The New High Protein Diet

The New High Protein Diet

C.V. Clark

Vermilion
LONDON

7 9 10 8 6

First published in 2002 by Vermilion,
an imprint of Ebury Press, Random House,
20 Vauxhall Bridge Road, London SW1V 2SA
www.randomhouse.co.uk

Random House Australia (Pty) Limited
20 Alfred Street, Milsons Point, Sydney,
New South Wales 2061, Australia

Random House New Zealand Limited
18 Poland Road, Glenfield, Auckland 10, New Zealand

Random House South Africa (Pty) Limited
Endulini, 5a Jubilee Road, Parktown 2193, South Africa

The Random House Group Limited Reg. No. 954009

Papers used by Vermilion are natural, recyclable products made from wood grown in sustainable forests.

Printed and bound in Great Britain by Bookmarque Ltd, Croydon, Surrey

A CIP catalogue record for this book is available from the British Library.

ISBN 0 09 188426 8

The advice offered in this book is not intended to be a substitute for the advice and counsel of your personal physician. Always consult a medical practitioner before embarking on a diet, or a course of exercise. Neither the author nor the publisher can be held responsible for any loss or claim arising out of the use, or misuse, of the suggestions made, or the failure to take medical advice.

Contents

Part III: How to Exercise – Without Really Trying 235

Acknowledgements

I would like to thank my wife for her patience, understanding, support and considerable advice, without which
the book would not have been possible; my young son,
David, for his occasional patience and understanding; and
my young daughter, Heather, for her total lack of patience
with her father, with the result that life is many things but
never boring!

Further information on this diet can be obtained on:
www.charlesclark.uk.com.

Preface

A completely new approach to dieting

Most people want to lose some weight, but the problem is that it really is hard to achieve – until now! This system is not a diet as such, it's a completely new way of enjoying food while programming your body medically to lose fat. So it's easy. All you have to do is follow some very simple rules, and you will automatically lose excess fat at the fastest safe rate for the body. And you will be enjoying absolutely delicious food in almost unlimited quantities. The desire to be slimmer is all you need to achieve your goal – or to put it another way, it's all I need to make sure you do! This system works for everyone, whether you want to lose a few pounds or a lot of pounds, because you are programming your body (not manipulating it with an abnormal diet regime), and it will automatically reduce your weight to the correct level for you, and stop. You can be absolutely certain that if you follow this medically based diet, you will lose your fat quickly, easily and without pain (and especially without hunger pains). You don't need superhuman willpower, endless amounts of time to prepare complex low-calorie recipes, or an unlimited bank balance to afford expensive pre-packaged diet foods. You definitely don't ever need to be hungry – and this doesn't mean you have to be constantly munching on lettuce and cottage cheese to stave off the agony of hunger pains (it doesn't work anyway, as all experienced dieters know).

Seriously, you can and will lose fat (not just weight) easily and effectively by adhering to a diet determined by established medical facts. Your body is already programmed to burn its own fat under certain conditions (and I don't mean starvation, in which the body actually breaks down protein in addition to fat). This diet will show you how you can easily programme your body to burn fat without exercise, and how you can keep the weight off without ever counting calories again.

To be successful, a diet must:

Get rid of excess fat

'Fat', not 'weight'. You want to look slimmer, not just weigh less. The difference is important, as I will explain on pages 238–91.

Allow you to live a normal life while losing the fat

There is no point in a diet taking over your life. If you have previously subscribed to the 'No pain, no gain' school of dieting, you may be surprised to learn that this really needn't be the case. Similarly, there is no point in advocating a diet in which hours every day are devoted to the preparation of complex meals; most people don't have that much spare time.

The diet must work quickly – the fat must disappear!

Well, I can't make the fat disappear overnight, but I can make it disappear quite quickly. Certainly fast enough to retain your interest in persevering. It is human nature to be impatient for results when dieting, especially if the diet is uncomfortable (as almost all are). You need results, and fast!

The diet must not be too expensive

Once again, there is no point in producing an effective diet if no-one can afford it. Unfortunately, junk food is inexpensive because it's just that – junk. Remember, your body is your most important possession. If you give it rubbish, it stops working.

The diet must be practical

It can't take up too much time. The people at most risk of succumbing to fast (and therefore fattening) food are those in full-time jobs. Unfortunately, no diet can compete for speed with pre-packaged foods, but if you can take just a little time out of your busy schedule to prepare the meals, you will be rewarded with the body you want, not the one that pre-packaged food has given you. And as an added bonus you will be healthier, fitter and much more self-confident.

You must not be hungry

The dieter's nightmare – literally. On the majority of diets, the agitated dieter lives in the cheerless world of counting calories, constant pangs of hunger and daily guilt complexes over some minor dietary indiscretion – not to mention the torture of constantly thinking about food. *On this diet you will not be hungry*: your appetite will be satisfied by good food, and you will be very satisfied with the results.

The diet must not allow blood sugar to become low

Low blood sugar (hypoglycaemia) is the most common cause of the behaviour pattern I have termed the 'diet syndrome': tiredness, fatigue, irritability, mood swings and irrational actions. It's not just because you're weak and hungry from lack of food, it's because your blood sugar is low. In fact, it's all perfectly rational: when your blood sugar is low, the brain does not function properly (because brain cells use sugar for energy) and therefore you experience all of the symptoms described. This must not be allowed to happen, or the diet will inevitably fail. Eventually you feel so weak you need to have some sugar – usually sweets or a cake – and the downward spiral begins again. And finally:

The diet must maintain the weight loss

As you all know, many 'starvation' diets (because that's what they are) are initially successful, but soon afterwards you regain all of the fat, usually with interest! So after suffering all that pain and discomfort, a few months later (or even less) you're back to square one. And to cap it all, you are convinced it must be your fault for not sticking to the diet. In fact, as I'll explain, it *isn't* your fault; the weight would have come back anyway, because you haven't lost fat, you've lost protein.

The diet expounded in this book won't do that. You will lose weight easily, and the weight you lose will actually be body fat, so you will achieve your goal. And if you continue to follow some simple principles in your diet after finally ridding yourself of the fat, it will never come back.

In summary, you need a diet which:

- stimulates your body to burn its own fat (instead of muscle protein, as in many diets)
- doesn't cost too much
- doesn't take too much time for preparation

- ✪ acts very quickly to cause loss of body fat (while completely satisfying your appetite, and actually being very tasty)
- ✪ does not cause any of the distressing symptoms of low blood sugar usually associated with dieting.

And the fat must not come back! Impossible? No, it's not impossible, it's not even difficult. It's actually quite easy, as you will see. But first, we have to examine the principles of most calorie-control diets to understand their strengths and weaknesses – and especially to understand why almost all are doomed to failure. It really is very important to understand why other diets don't work, so that you never make the same mistake again. It's also important to understand the fundamental basis of dieting the *medical* way – which is truly very simple – because you can then take control of your own body . . . And no-one else is as interested in your body as YOU!

Go ahead, take the plunge and start now. You will see real weight loss in the first two weeks, and you will feel much better. Enjoy your new body, which is the real you, without the unwanted pounds.

PART I

The New High Protein Diet

The New High Protein Diet will change your life if you're overweight, because you will lose weight quickly, easily and painlessly, and – providing you keep to some very simple guidelines – the weight will not return. Part I of the book explains the basic principles of the diet. It is really essential to read this because when you *understand* the problem it's much easier to solve. And being overweight *is* a medical problem, it's *not* just a question of eating too much, which is the usual explanation given (and which is completely incorrect). It's an imbalance of hormones; in fact, our present high-carbohydrate diet actually stimulates certain hormones to deposit fat. Part I of the book will explain how you can easily *reverse* this process, making the hormones *remove* your body fat preferentially, *despite enjoying a high-calorie diet.* You will be able to eat delicious foods and never be hungry, whilst losing weight at the safest rate for the human body. And you will probably be eating the most nutritious food in your life, as this diet is specially designed to incorporate all of the essential nutrition for health – unlike many other diets. The New High Protein Diet is really a way of life, rather than a diet, in which you re-programme your body to lose weight, and the hormones do the work for you. And the way you re-programme the system is simply by eating certain combinations of healthy foods and avoiding others. It really is that simple. With the correct advice, anyone can lose weight easily and painlessly, so let's begin.

Chapter 1

How *Not* to Diet

The reason I am explaining how not to diet is that most
people have being going about losing weight in the wrong
way for years, and I am firmly of the opinion that to lose
weight successfully you need to understand why previous
diets have failed and why this new diet *will* work.

Studies have shown that less than 5 per cent of people
are successful in permanently losing weight on a diet. To
put this another way, 95 per cent of dieters fail to lose
weight for any significant period of time – most eventually
gaining more weight than they had before they started to
diet. As all of these people have a real desire to be slimmer,
they try another diet, and another one, and so it goes on.
And as all of them are serious dieters, a billion-dollar
industry develops to service their needs, which is self-
sustaining as 95 per cent of the diets fail. This is not
intended as a criticism of the diet industry; on the contrary,
being slimmer is undoubtedly healthier for most
individuals (apart from those with an unrealistic self-image)
and therefore a slimmer, healthier body is definitely to be
encouraged.

Where most diets go wrong

The problem with the majority of diets is that, without
superhuman willpower, the dieter cannot sustain the
regime. This is down to a variety of reasons:

Hunger

A constant aggravating hunger, with the usual mood swings and irritability caused by low blood sugar, is enough to drive anyone to the nearest fast-food outlet.

Preparation time

Hours to prepare – diet fails! How many times have you read 'Preparation time 15 minutes', and two hours later you're still chopping the broccoli?

Cost

Dietary ingredients often cost a small fortune. Little wonder that so many people opt for the frozen pizza: nutritionally disastrous but cheap.

Boring repetition

There are only so many ways to prepare a lettuce leaf.

Polystyrene taste

A rice cake tastes like a rice cake no matter how many times you try to convince yourself otherwise.

And when (not 'if') the diet fails, we are convinced it must be our fault, because, after all, it can't take much willpower to achieve, as we have constant reminders in slimming magazines of 'ordinary' (usually grossly overweight) people who apparently slimmed from 25 to 10 stones without any difficulty at all. So now not only are we unhappy about our weight and appearance, but we are also guilty about our abject failure to lose the fat. What can be so difficult when we have detailed instructions from eminent experts – or even better, the advice of celebrity dieters who seem to lose weight with no problem at all? Of course, the benefits of unlimited free time and money to spend on improving their physical appearance may contribute to their success!

Let us deal with each of these points in turn, because if we can't clear up the mental problem, the physical problem will remain. Most importantly, you have nothing to feel guilty about! You are not a failure, and you are not wrong. The diets are virtually unworkable for almost everybody. How can I be so certain? Simple. Remember I said that current diets failed to achieve sustained weight loss in 95 per cent of cases? As an experienced medical researcher, I can assure you that if an event occurs in 95 per cent of the population, it is considered normal by scientists, and if it occurs in 5 per cent of the population, it is considered abnormal. So, without any doubt, to succeed on present diets is definitely abnormal in scientific terms. In other words, *you* are normal, it's the diet that's not!

How can this be? We are bombarded with constant information regarding the need to reduce our calories; consume less fat, red meat and eggs; eat more vegetables and fruit, and so on. The list is seemingly endless, and we are told that if we do this we will be slimmer and healthier. This is true up to a point, but the problem is that for the majority of people it is a very difficult eating pattern to implement – and worse, it will *not* cause loss of body fat in the majority of circumstances.

Loss of fat medically involves adjusting the *balance* of the various food groups in the diet, not just reducing calories. Unfortunately, loss of body fat is not a simple equation whereby if you reduce your intake of food, you will inevitably lose fat. You won't. All experienced dieters will be familiar with the shock and anger of staring at the non-moving bathroom scales, even though they have eaten virtually nothing. It is balance, not quantity, that makes a diet work. And this makes life much easier for everyone, as you can easily keep to the diet when you find food satisfying, and you feel well, especially when there are no restrictions on the quantities of many tasty foods.

In many instances, when you reduce your intake of food, you lose body protein (especially muscle). So while your body shape may appear smaller, and your waist measurement may decrease, *the amount of body fat remains virtually the same*. What's more, as the underlying layer of body fat is only slightly reduced, when you relinquish your starvation diet and resume eating (even moderately), the body proteins are the first to be reformed by the body, so you rapidly increase in weight (and girth), because protein is twice as heavy as fat. The classic failed diet! So you see, *you* didn't fail, the diet was doomed to failure from the start.

So we arrive at the next obvious question: why bother? If all diets are doomed to failure (or involve intense pain and suffering), there doesn't appear to be much point. Well there is! First, all diets are not doomed to failure, it is only the way in which the diet is *applied* that is unworkable. And second, I can assure you that you will *definitely* lose body fat (not just weight, but actually the fat that you really want to lose) on this diet – easily, painlessly, with little effort or expense, and almost enjoyably. This seems too good to be true, but I can assure you that it is true, as you will see. As an experienced Consultant Surgeon, I am not given to exaggeration; just the facts, pure and simple.

A diet that works

But first of all it is essential to explain the basics of dieting in simple, straightforward terms. Having practised medicine for over twenty years, I am sure that the only way to achieve success in any form of treatment is for patients to be fully informed about their conditions. And let us be perfectly clear about this: being overweight *is* a medical condition, and should be treated as such. Apart from the possible physical problems of obesity (hypertension, heart disease, diabetes, arthritis), the mental distress must be taken seriously: if we are unhappy, our stress levels increase exponentially, and that is a real problem for our ultimate health and well-being.

To the facts of nutrition. Be sure to read this section carefully – it is quite simple to understand – because if you don't fully grasp the principles of the diet, you won't get it right. The first point to make is that you won't be counting calories any more. You are going to adhere to certain rules in choosing foods, which will enable the fat to be 'burned off' (a term I dislike, but it conveys the meaning excellently) by the body. So you will have immense freedom to choose a wide variety of foods *in virtually unlimited quantities*. For the first time, you will eat well while dieting. I know this sounds like some 'never to be repeated offer' on television, but it is based on established medical principles, and does work.

You've probably read some of the following facts before (and almost certainly if you are an experienced dieter) but please read them again, because the subsequent paragraphs will definitely be new to most readers, and form the basis of the diet. Once you understand the principles, you will be able to apply them easily – and successfully.

As most people know, there are five basic food groups that we require: carbohydrates, fats, proteins, vitamins and minerals. The first three (carbohydrates, fats and proteins) give us energy; proteins also provide amino acids, the building blocks of the body. Vitamins and minerals are absolutely essential for the efficient maintenance of body functions (like chemical reactions), but vitamins and minerals *do not* provide energy, and therefore – provided we ensure our diet is not deficient in these essential elements – vitamins and minerals are not part of the weight-loss equation. So, we are left with carbohydrates, fats and protein. The secret of burning body fat lies in the relative proportion of these constituents in the diet.

There are three golden rules that you must understand to diet effectively:

1. *Your body does not work like a machine*

What does this mean? Let me explain – because this is the reason for the failure of low-calorie diets. The way that scientists determine the energy content (or 'calories') of any given food is literally to burn the food in an instrument, like a type of mini-oven that measures the heat produced. Heat is the way in which energy is 'released' when a material burns, and we give the food a 'caloric content' depending on how much heat is generated. For example, 1 gram of fat produces about 9 calories, whereas 1 gram of carbohydrate or protein produces about 4 calories. Seems fairly simple. On this basis, you might reasonably assume that fat in your diet (as it has twice as many calories as protein or carbohydrate) has twice as much risk of being deposited as fat in your body.

In fact this is wrong. The human body does not function

like a machine, and it does not burn food in the same way as a laboratory instrument, so the simple calculation of calories based upon the relative amounts of carbohydrates, proteins and fats is fundamentally flawed. As you will see, by applying medical principles to the way your body processes food, you will be able to eat *more* calories than someone on a low-calorie diet, and yet *you* will lose body fat and they will not. The absorption of food in the gut depends upon a complex series of interactions, which means that by varying the composition of your food, you can eat far more calories (and calories of tasty foods rather than the usual tasteless foods) and lose weight, while someone else may eat fewer calories without losing any weight. Incredible, but true! Now you may begin to see why so many years are wasted counting calories and yet not losing weight – or fat.

2. *Fats in your diet do not necessarily cause weight gain*

In other words, although fat has double the calorie content of carbohydrate or protein, it does not necessarily cause you to put on twice as much weight. If your diet is properly balanced, you can include a moderate (not excessive) amount of fat in your diet *and actually lose weight.* Once again, this is based upon the fact that the body does not function simply as a machine. This is not intended to encourage you to consume excessive amounts of fats, but rather to eat 'healthy' fats in moderation. In association with the remainder of the programme, you will then lose far more weight (and especially fat) than you ever did counting calories – and with very little effort, you will keep the weight off.

Remember, certain fats are essential components of the

human body. (No, I don't mean the bulges over your tummy and hips; we'll get rid of those.) Essential fats make up the outer coating of nerve cells and form the basis of many hormones in the body – including the sex hormones. We need these lipids (a medical term for fats), but not the fat cells deposited in all the wrong places. So you can see that some fats are absolutely essential for a healthy body. You can eat certain fats in your diet, and at the same time remove the unsightly bulges of storage fat around your waist and hips, as this diet will clearly demonstrate. In other words, not all fats are bad.

3. *You can programme your body to burn excess body fat instead of dietary calories*

This is the most amazing statement of all – the 'Holy Grail' for all dieters. You can programme your body to burn its own fat – especially from the waist and hip region – in preference to the food you consume. In other words, you can have your figurative cake, and eat it.

How can this be possible? Like most of medicine, it's actually very simple, as I'll explain in the next chapter. This information forms the basis of everything that follows. Please take the time to understand it, because you do have to follow the rules of the diet exactly for it to be successful. Once you understand the principles, you will be able to keep to the diet easily, and then you can proceed to eat your way to losing fat.

Chapter 2

How the New High Protein Diet Works

To understand the way in which this diet effectively 'burns' excess body fat, we must first of all examine the three main energy foods in our diet and, in particular, their effects on the body when they are digested and absorbed.

The carbohydrate cycle

Carbohydrates are – in simple terms – sugars and starches. They are absorbed from the digestive tract reasonably quickly, which is the reason why we get a rapid energy boost from a bar of chocolate or a pastry. But – and this is the important part – when our blood sugar levels go up, a hormone called insulin is released, which then starts to lower the blood sugar level very quickly. When the sugar level in our blood goes down rapidly, we feel weak and faint ('hypoglycaemia' is medicalspeak for low blood sugar), so we have another sweet food to boost our sugar level. Again, we feel better for a while, and then insulin kicks in to lower our blood sugar and make us feel weak once more. And so the cycle goes on. Most people associate insulin with diabetes, in which there is a problem with insulin production, but actually insulin is an essential hormone in everyone. Your body simply can't cope with too much sugar in the diet.

The Carbohydrate Cycle

Eating refined carbohydrates   →   More insulin

    ↑   ↓

Hunger/irritability   ←   Lower blood sugar
                                                (hypoglycaemia)

Every dieter reading this chapter has probably experienced these symptoms. Even worse than the constant ups and downs in energy levels are the difficult mood swings that accompany the energy fluctuations. And every time we have another cake or chocolate – which we really must have or suffer the discomfort of low blood sugar, which nobody can ignore I can assure you – the pounds pile on.

Just when you thought it couldn't get worse, it does! Insulin has many essential functions in maintaining life, but it has one very bad action for the dieter: *it causes excess carbohydrate to be stored as fat*. In other words, it actually stimulates the deposit of fat around our bodies.

Let us go over this again, just to be certain that you fully understand the mechanism of fat storage in the body, because by shutting down this mechanism, you reverse the process: instead of making fat, you burn fat.

- When you are hungry, you eat carbohydrates, which provide a rapid source of energy.

- This stimulates the production of insulin by the body, which quickly lowers the blood sugar, making you

feel weak and irritable, so you eat more
carbohydrates to make you feel better, which it does –
but only briefly.

- Insulin then stimulates the deposit of excess
carbohydrate as fat, especially around the waist and
hips. Even worse, it actually prevents body fat from
being used to provide energy, so you can never break
down body fat if insulin levels are elevated.

The Effects of Insulin

INSULIN

↙   ↘

Lower blood sugar   Converts sugar to
                                 Body fat

↓

Hunger

Breaking the cycle

How can you put an end to this vicious circle? If you don't
eat, you become weaker and weaker (and more irritable),
as you all know. The answer is simple:

Reduce the insulin!

If you decrease the amount of insulin your body releases,
your blood glucose levels won't plummet so dramatically,

so you won't become weak and irritable, and you won't feel the need to eat more carbohydrate for energy. Ultimately, therefore, you won't deposit the fat on your waist and hips.

Even better, if you lower your insulin levels, the body's mechanisms are actually directed to burn body fat preferentially. In other words, you have switched on the body's automatic fat-burning mechanism. Just one small problem. How exactly do you achieve this minor miracle of lowering the insulin level, and therefore converting to 'fat-burning' mode (instead of the usual 'fat-deposit' mode)? Once again, the answer is very simple:

Reduce your intake of refined carbohydrates

Low carbohydrate diet causes *breakdown* of body fat

Reduce refined
carbohydrates

↓

Lower insulin level

↙   ↘

No fat deposited   Breakdown of body fat

The production of insulin is essentially controlled by

carbohydrate intake, not fats or proteins, so if you cut down drastically on refined carbohydrates, your insulin levels reduce naturally, and you start to burn body fat. It really is that easy.

All of a sudden, you can now clearly see why previous diets have failed. Almost all diets instruct you to *increase* your daily intake of carbohydrates, usually as cereals, grains, pasta, rice and pulses (peas and beans). Even if you reduce your calorie intake to below the level you need each day, unless you switch off the insulin (and convert to the mode of burning body fat) there is always the tendency to deposit some of the food as more fat. That is what insulin does, and insulin is stimulated by carbohydrates. So you weren't a failure after all, it just was not medically possible to lose weight safely on some of the diets you followed. The system for burning fat was switched off.

Reduce carbohydrate – not calories – to lose weight

Identical calorie intake

↙   ↘

Low carbohydrate diet   High carbohydrate diet

↓   ↓

Weight loss   Weight gain

Of course, we certainly do not want to switch off our insulin completely; we need insulin, but our bodies do not need, and were never designed to cope with, large quantities of refined carbohydrates, such as the immense loads of refined sugars and starches in the pre-packaged foods that form the basis of the modern Western diet. If we cut out the foods that our bodies cannot safely tolerate, insulin production returns to its normal level, we burn any excess fat and return to our normal shape. You don't see fat animals in nature, because animals don't eat our diet.

There is one other very important point that is going to become quite obvious in a moment. If you switch on your automatic fat-burning mechanism by cutting out refined carbohydrates and sugars, what else do you have to restrict in the diet? NOTHING! Yes, that's right, your eyes are not deceiving you: there are absolutely no other restrictions in the diet. You can eat virtually as much as you like of any other foods, and you will still lose fat. This is hard to believe, but true. For the first time, you are using the body's own established mechanisms to lose fat. So you are *not* going to be hungry, or irritable, or spend all of your time counting calories, and as you will be eating a diet high in protein, vitamins and minerals, your body will be receiving healthy nutrition while losing fat.

Chapter 3

The Principles of the
New High Protein Diet

This diet is the most effective way of losing body fat. Remember, if we go on a starvation diet (which is all that many so-called diets are), we lose *weight* but not much *fat*. In starvation mode, we use up our energy stores of carbohydrate first (in the form of a substance called glycogen). However, the body can store only a little glycogen, and this is used up within two days. Then we start breaking down fat and protein. But we can't afford to lose body proteins: our muscle mass decreases, we become noticeably weaker, and our immunity is compromised because the lack of protective immunoglobulin proteins means we are subject to an increased risk of infection. Not good!

Sure, we look slimmer (because our body shape *under* the fat layer is smaller), and we certainly weigh less (because muscle is much heavier than fat), but we are weaker and becoming unhealthy. There is no point in dieting if it's going to make us ill. And, of course, because we need our muscles, when we even slightly stray from the diet, our bodies immediately rebuild muscle and we regain all of the 'lost' weight very quickly. Yet another diet fails – because it was never going to work in the first place. And we have succeeded in making ourselves considerably less healthy in the process. Not only have we gone through a period of reduced immunity and a lack of proteins, minerals, vitamins, antioxidants and other essential nutrients, there is evidence that so-called 'yo-yo' dieting of this nature is detrimental to health in the longer term.

Unlike calorie-control diets, the New High Protein Diet will work, and it is very easy to implement

Quite simply, we are going to virtually eliminate all refined carbohydrates and sugars (which are also carbohydrates), leaving us with a low-carbohydrate, high-protein diet. Of course, you may have heard of (and probably tried) high-protein diets before, and they all failed *because the carbohydrates were not restricted*. Remember, unless you switch off the mechanism to make fat, and switch on the mechanism to burn fat, it is very difficult to lose body fat. On this diet, you will be cutting out virtually all refined carbohydrates (which your body does not need) so that body fat is burned preferentially, to provide energy.

What are refined carbohydrates?

Sugar, starch, white flour, cakes, bread, pasta and rice are the usual culprits. These foods have very little nutritional value and, what's more, can cause medical and fat problems. Of course, there are forms of these carbohydrates – such as wholemeal rice, wholemeal bread and wholemeal pasta – that do have nutritional benefits and which you can reintroduce later, but in the initial stage of the diet, you have to reduce *all* carbohydrates, to switch on the fat-burning mechanism.

Everything containing refined carbohydrates is excluded

A list of foods containing refined carbohydrates can be found on pages 271–4 but you should definitely cut out all pasta, rice, cakes and biscuits, and stick to a maximum of one slice of bread per day. Your body will rapidly adjust to a healthy, high-protein, low-carbohydrate diet, and will burn body fat. The bottom line is that you don't need refined carbohydrates and processed sugars. These foods provide energy (which you can easily obtain from better sources) and no other form of essential nutrition – and when you eat more than the energy you can use immediately, the rest is stored as fat.

One point to be aware of is that refined carbohydrates can appear in many unexpected sources. You probably know that bread, cakes, pastries, biscuits, pies, pizzas, potato crisps and fried potato chips all contain refined carbohydrates, but pasta, rice, most breakfast cereals, most tinned foods, many pre-packaged foods, tinned vegetables, tinned soups, and prepared sauces do as well . . . In fact, the list goes on and on. Virtually all 'fast foods' contain very high proportions of refined carbohydrates – as well as hydrogenated fats – and if your diet is high in refined carbohydrates and hydrogenated fats, you will definitely put on weight.

If you're worried that by cutting out refined carbohydrates you'll have virtually no foods left to choose from, fear not. In fact, high-protein and nutritious foods such as meat, poultry, fish, shellfish and eggs are all open to you, along with vegetables, cheese, spices and herbs, from which you can easily produce delicious, healthy and quick meals. You'll be relieved to hear that you don't have to live on a diet of lettuce and tomato (nutritious as they are, they are rather limited in taste on their own). On the contrary, you will be eating virtually *limitless* quantities of very tasty food, complemented by delicious sauces and dressings: in other words, real food! To demonstrate just how easily this can be achieved, a comprehensive list of recipes is included in Part II of the book, all of which can easily be incorporated into your busy lifestyle. In short, you'll eat well and still lose fat.

What about fats in your diet? I've advised you to cut out refined carbohydrates and eat a high-protein diet, but what about the amount of fat you consume? This is going to seem a strange thing to say, and it's against all of the dietary advice you've been given in the past, but if you follow the principles of this diet carefully, *you don't need worry about how much fat you're consuming.* No, I have not gone mad, and I'm certainly not advocating a high-fat diet, but most of the 'bad' fats are actually integrated into the sugary, starchy foods you have already excluded, and you will naturally avoid them when you stop eating these foods. So by excluding the refined carbohydrates, you have excluded the 'bad' fats from your diet at a single stroke.

Not all fats are bad

Some fats are actually essential for life. We need fats to make part of the outer walls around cells in the body (of which there are trillions), to produce the sheaths of nerve cells, and to make hormones that are essential for life. In addition, certain essential vitamins are fat-soluble, which means that you need fat to absorb them. I'm not, of course, suggesting that you will be healthier on a diet of burgers and French fries (which you have just excluded from your diet anyway), but the flip side of the coin is that you also will not be healthy without essential fats in your diet. The secret is knowing which are the essential fats (which incidentally have the most taste) and which are the ones to avoid. Most 'fast' foods are cooked in 'trans' fats, which are definitely not good for your health.

The old story that if you eat fat you will get fat is only true if you *also* eat carbohydrates. If you don't eat carbohydrates, you will switch off the fat-making process to a large extent, and fats in the diet do not switch it on. So you can eat more fats of the correct type in these circumstances, without weight gain, and actually mobilise your own excess body fat in the process.

Fats in our diet, apart from being essential for many body functions, also play an important role in digestion. They *slow* the absorption process in the intestine, preventing the highs and lows of blood sugar levels produced by carbohydrates and insulin, so we feel more stable and have less acute mood swings. Fats in the diet make us feel satisfied after a meal, preventing the hunger pangs that are experienced within an hour or two of a carbohydrate-based meal. And finally, the body tells us when to stop eating 'pure' fats (unlike the fats combined with sugars in, for example, cakes and chocolate, which can be quite addictive). In fact, we only overindulge in fats when they are combined with sugars or starches (such as in potato chips). I have never heard of a case of overeating associated purely with butter, cheese, avocados, fresh nuts, eggs, or animal or fish products. On the contrary, many natural oils are healthy. An excellent example is fish oils, which have been clearly proven to be very good for us – and no-one ever heard of a fat fish! Personally, I do not particularly like the taste of excess animal fat, so I would still recommend lean meat; the amount of saturated fat in a lean cut of meat is certainly not excessive.

So you can clearly see that if you cut out refined

carbohydrates from your diet, you simultaneously exclude most of the 'bad' fats, lose body fat, feel better, look better, and actually get significantly healthier – without being hungry or tired. What could be easier?

A two-step programme

What? No bread or pasta or cakes or rice, for ever! No more chips, or burgers, or steak pies? It's not worth living; I can hear the storm of protest from some of you already. No, don't worry. You don't have to forsake all of these culinary delights forever. Remember, this is a fat reduction diet. You have to get rid of the excess fat that you have accumulated over the years, so obviously you have to avoid fattening foods at the moment, but you can eat them at a later stage *in moderation*. Your first goal is to remove the causes of fat accumulation in the first place, but once you have lost your excess fat (and it will go faster than you expect on this diet) then you can include some of these desirable (if unhealthy) foods, but in much smaller proportions than before. I'm not suggesting that you never again eat cake or ice cream – just not during the diet!

In essence, this means that there are two stages to the diet: a weight loss stage and a weight maintenance stage. In the first stage (weight loss), you have to keep strictly to the 40–60 gram daily limit for carbohydrates to lose weight quickly. When you have reached your target size, or when the weight loss has stopped (which is your body telling you that this is the correct weight for you and you won't lose any more weight safely), you can increase your carbohydrate intake again, in moderation (the weight maintenance stage). Your body will quickly tell you if you're eating too much carbohydrate, because you'll gain weight. The amount of carbohydrate really is different for everyone, but you'll almost certainly be able to eat more than 60 grams per day without weight gain.

In effect, this simply means that after you have lost weight, providing you eat refined carbohydrates in moderation, you will not gain weight as fat. But I can assure you that after you have re-programmed your body on this healthy, satisfying diet, you will no longer be addicted to sugar and starchy foods – because that is what this is, a mild form of addiction which your body has developed in response to fluctuating sugar levels and the associated fluctuating insulin levels.

After only a few days on this diet, you will find that you are not as hungry as before, not only because you are eating sufficient amounts to stave off hunger, but also because you have literally re-programmed your body to a more normal desire for food. This is a natural consequence of a high-protein, low-carbohydrate diet. In many cases, individuals find that they still enjoy carbohydrates after the diet, but they no longer need them in such large quantities. The diet is effective in the longer term because your eating patterns are re-set. You no longer have to think about what you must not eat; the intense desire is no longer there, so it's easy to resist. Many people find they have simply lost the taste for the 'bad' foods, which makes keeping slim so much easier.

It is much easier to prevent the fat from re-accumulating after this diet, because you have actually lost most of your excess fat in the first place. As you now appreciate, calorie-control seldom works in actually losing fat, because the mechanism for fat storage has not been switched off. So you can return to some of your old ways, and if you only eat the 'bad' foods in moderation, you probably won't put on weight.

A new sense of well-being

You will have noticed that I continually use the term 'fat' instead of 'weight'. There are two reasons for this: firstly, the weight you are losing is actually fat on this diet, unlike the loss of weight as body protein on other diets; and secondly, the word 'fat' is very emotive. It embodies the feeling of dislike (almost disgust) that the dieter feels towards this excess tissue. Instead of disguising this unpleasant feeling with inaccurate terms like 'weight loss', I believe that the most important step is to accept the problem at face value – physically, psychologically, and emotionally. There are few more emotive subjects in Western society than body fat.

On this diet, you will re-educate your body to accept and enjoy healthier food, which actually tastes better, because you will be shown how easy it is and how good you feel. And this second point is very important: you *will* feel better. Not just because you have succeeded in losing fat and you look much better, but also because you will be – and feel – healthier. You will be able to return to a much less restricted diet after you have lost the fat you wanted to lose, because the fat has gone, whereas on previous diets the fat was still there, merely disguised by the slimming effects of loss of muscle and body protein.

But to rid yourself of excess body fat is not enough. My aim is to ensure that you are much healthier, and that is why the diet is divided into two stages:

- In the early stage – excess weight-loss phase – you

concentrate on getting rid of the fat. Carbohydrates *must* be severely restricted in this phase for effective and rapid weight loss.

- In the later stage – the weight-maintenance phase – when you are satisfied with your weight, you are allowed a much more liberal diet, because it's much more difficult to gain weight (as fat) when you exclude most of the refined carbohydrates. This means that you can eat far more foods than you ever thought possible, remain healthy, and not deposit additional adipose tissue (medicalspeak for fat).

Losing weight safely

It is very important that you do not reduce in size too quickly. I know everyone wants to lose the fat as quickly as possible – and this diet will work quite rapidly – but you shouldn't try to accelerate the effect of the diet by reducing the amounts you eat. This is a common mistake among dieters, and will lead to inevitable failure. This diet will reduce weight – as fat – *at the most efficient rate for your body*. It is much faster than other diets, and it results in definite loss of fat (and not protein) if followed correctly. But if you tamper with the rules, it won't work, because it depends entirely upon switching off the fat-storage mechanisms in the body. For example, if you add in one or two cakes, or biscuits, or bars of chocolate, this diet will fail because your carbohydrate intake will be too high. It is also important that you do not reduce your weight too rapidly because:

- It is not healthy, and can make you very sick, with

reduced immunity from infection. This high-protein diet will ensure that does not happen.

- If you lose weight too quickly, your skin doesn't have enough time to adapt to the new, smaller you, and you will be left with unsightly folds of excess skin.

How many times have you read of dieters requiring surgery after severe dieting? It is obviously ridiculous to require surgery – and have surgical scars and possible post-operative complications – as a result of a diet that was intended to make you look more attractive! If you reduce in size at a regular pace – usually 1–1.5 kilos per week initially – you will achieve a much better final cosmetic appearance, which is the aim of the diet. By restricting refined carbohydrates, you will lose weight steadily *and at the fastest rate your body can withstand while still remaining healthy*. More importantly, you will continue to lose weight at a rate of about 1 kilo per week until you approach the 'normal' weight for your height and shape, which is genetically pre-programmed in all of us from birth. At this point, weight loss will slow down – in other words, your genes determine your normal shape, as long as you supply your body with the necessary nutrition in the correct proportions. The mechanism is already in place: you just have to provide the building blocks and your genes will do the rest.

Chapter 4

Eating for Health

Healthy eating implies boring, tasteless food: salad (again) without vinaigrette, plain vegetables, and fat-free (therefore taste-free) meals. This chapter will completely destroy this myth, demonstrating that delicious food can also be healthy. It will explain why this diet is made up the way it is, why certain foods are included and others are excluded: in essence, why it works, and why you can't break the rules and still be successful. If you take the time to read this chapter (and re-read it later), you will understand what you have to do – and why – and you will start to take control of your own health. That is the whole point of the book. It is not just to lose weight (as fat), but also to be fitter and healthier, feel better, have more self-confidence, and enjoy your life so much more. While losing your fat, you will achieve all these other goals without even trying. But you will find it much easier to stick to the programme if you understand how it works, rather than just following it blindly.

In Chapter 1, I briefly discussed the major essential components in our diet: proteins, fats, carbohydrates, vitamins and minerals. Here I will elaborate on the essential functions of each of these food groups, focusing a little bit on their main actions in keeping us healthy, how we can burn our body fat by altering the various proportions of these groups in the diet, and at the same time not only maintain our health but actually improve it.

During this diet, no-one will feel hungry or deprived –

apart, perhaps, from totally addicted chocaholics, and even they can return to a decreased level of addiction after they have lost most of their unwanted kilos.

Proteins

These are the building blocks of the body. Or, to be more accurate, proteins are made up of amino acids, which are the building blocks of the body. Every protein is constructed of many amino acids, and when we eat foods containing protein, our digestive system breaks down the protein into its component amino acids, and our body then joins them together again as the structural proteins we need, a little like a human Lego set.

Amino acids – the building blocks of life

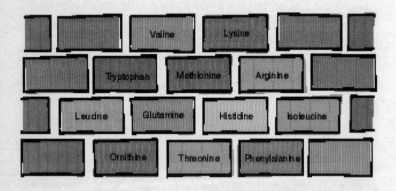

Proteins are essential for building not only the structures we can see – like skin, bones, hair and nails – but also all the myriad tissues we can't see but which keep us alive, like the blood cells, immune system, nervous system and chemicals that make reactions occur, called enzymes. The bottom line is, we need certain proteins for life.

Although all of the proteins we require can be supplied from plant sources, 'complete' proteins (which means they contain all of the essential amino acids we need) come primarily from animal sources: beef, pork, fish, poultry, and eggs. So animal sources of protein will form the basis of this diet for two main reasons: firstly, they will supply all of the essential amino acids to prevent protein deficiencies (which are very serious), and secondly, it is much more complicated to ensure that you obtain all of the necessary amino acids from plants, especially for the beginner.

To make things even easier, animal proteins (beef, pork, fish, poultry and eggs) have negligible amounts of carbohydrates, so they switch off the insulin mechanism and switch on the fat-burning system. But what about the fat, and calories, in these foods? Fats will be discussed in the next section, but suffice it to say that if you switch off the fat-storage mechanism, the fats you eat in your diet will not be deposited as fat in your body. In the same way, if you switch off the fat-storage mechanism, the calorie content of foods is irrelevant – so ignore it. When you have switched on the fat-burning mechanism, it doesn't matter how many calories you eat, you will not put on weight, and you will lose fat – medically.

Fats

Contrary to popular belief, all fats are *not* bad for you. Some are, but probably not the ones you expect. Let's put the fat myth into perspective. We need certain fats for life. Hard though it may be to accept – especially after years of indoctrination – I'm afraid it's not only untrue that all fat in the diet is bad for you, it's positively wrong. We need fats for many reasons: to build cell walls, construct sheaths around nerve cells, and form hormones (chemical messengers in the body), to name just a few essential roles of fats in the body.

Like proteins, fats are made up of their own building blocks (called fatty acids), and we need certain essential fatty acids to live. We also need some fat in our diet for the correct absorption of essential components of the diet. For example, some of the vitamins we need are *fat soluble*, which means they 'dissolve' in fats but not in water. No fat, no absorption of certain essential vitamins (this will be discussed in more detail later).

But all fats are not equal. Some are very good, some not so good. Essential fatty acids are usually divided into two groups: omega-3 and omega-6.

- Omega-3 fatty acids are found in oily fish (such as herring, mackerel, salmon, sardines and tuna), fish oils, egg yolks, nuts, nut oils, and certain vegetable oils (especially flaxseed).

- Omega-6 fatty acids are found in egg yolks, seeds and seed oils (in particular sunflower, safflower and sesame), whole grains, certain vegetables and vegetable oils. Omega 6 fatty acids are also present in evening primrose and borage oils.

A special mention must be made of olive oil, which has a high proportion of monounsaturated oils. Although it is not rich in *essential* fatty acids, it is incredibly healthy, not least because of its vitamin E, magnesium, and antioxidant content – especially polyphenols.

So, obviously, we are going to incorporate these fats into our diet. But we are not going to *add* them to the diet, we are going to *replace* certain of the other types of fat in the diet with these 'healthy' fats. For example, by cooking with olive oil, and eating fish, eggs and certain vegetables, we create a diet high in protein, essential fatty acids, vitamins, minerals, and antioxidants (more about these later), and yet with no refined carbohydrates. Simple!

But what about the fats? A large egg alone provides about 100 kilocalories! This must lead to fat deposition around our midriff, among other places, mustn't it?

Wrong again!

You will not gain weight (as fat) on this diet. You may increase your body protein (as muscle, which is obviously good for you), but you will still lose body fat. How can this be? Surely if you eat more calories than you need, you must gain weight? No, this is the fallacy of the calorie-control diet theory. As I briefly explained back in Chapter 1, the body is not a simple combustion engine. It functions by a very complex system of interactions, and if you switch off the fat-storage system (by reducing carbohydrates below a particular level), it will burn body fat even if you are eating more calories than you absolutely require – provided the extra calories are not carbohydrates. Extra fat intake when the body is in fat-burning mode is simply passed out of the body again (mostly in the urine), without being absorbed, and without being stored as fat. So you can see that provided you switch off the fat-storage mechanism, you can eat more fats without gaining weight.

I can easily prove the fallacy of the calorie-counting

system of dieting. Some people have a medical condition that leads to problems with the absorption of certain foods from the intestine. No matter how much they eat of those foods, none are absorbed into the body, and the patient gradually loses weight (and health) despite a high-calorie intake.

Basic fallacy of low-calorie diets

High calorie intake

↙   ↘

Absorbs food normally   Poor absorption of food

↓   ↓

Gains weight   Losing weight – despite high calorie intake – because *food not absorbed by body*

According to the calorie-counting theory of dieting, this high-calorie intake should mean that these patients gain weight. On the contrary, due to their inability to absorb food, they lose weight. The obvious conclusion from this evidence is that making decisions on health without taking into account the complex interactions that occur within the human body will inevitably result in major errors of judgement. The concept that simply restricting calories will cause fat loss is one such error. *The 95 per cent failure rate of this method proves it does not work.*

So by activating the fat-burning mechanism in the body, you will lose your body fat, even if you are ingesting more calories as fat or protein. And because you are eating the 'right' food, you will be healthier, fitter and slimmer.

Do not misinterpret the message of this chapter. It is not intended to advocate a high-fat diet. Although you are eating 'pure' fats, you will actually be eating *less* fat, because most of the 'bad' fats are incorporated in foods with refined sugars and carbohydrates (such as cakes, pastries, pizza, pies, processed and packaged foods, fast foods, crisps and chips), which you have excluded from your diet. Instead, you have replaced them with essential fatty acids in eggs, fish, vegetables and nuts, among others.

These foods are more than just 'fats', even 'essential fats'. They contain high-quality complete proteins, essential vitamins and minerals, and are major sources of antioxidants, which basically keep us healthy, prevent cancer and various other unpleasant medical conditions, and seriously help to prevent ageing. So before we complain about the dangerous aspects of these fats (and there is a considerable amount of controversy about exactly how dangerous certain fats in the diet are, with strong evidence to suggest that the 'all saturated fats are bad' theory has major flaws), let us also remember the considerable benefits that some very good fats provide for our health and well-being.

Carbohydrates

These provide energy, and little else. 'Refined' carbohydrates provide energy, and *nothing* else, apart from causing the increased production of insulin, which promotes fat storage and prevents the burning of body fat. It would seem fairly obvious to the most casual observer that we don't need refined carbohydrates in our lives, and therefore we are going to exclude them from our diets.

However, apart from refined sugar, carbohydrates are seldom 'pure', but rather mixed with other constituents in various foods. These can be in foods, also containing fats, that are bad for your health (for example chips, cakes, pizzas and so forth), or in foods that are good for you, such as vegetables. The carbohydrates in fresh vegetables are very different from those in refined foods. Fresh vegetables contain what are known as 'complex' carbohydrates, which means they are absorbed much more slowly and more evenly over a period of time, as opposed to the rapid absorption (and associated rapid release of insulin) which occurs with refined sugars. Of much more importance with regard to health, carbohydrates in fresh vegetables are incorporated with vitamins, minerals, proteins and fibre – all of which we need for survival. They are not associated with refined fats, only essential fatty acids (in some vegetables).

I hope you can see the pattern of healthy dieting emerging. It is not about avoiding all fats and eating smaller amounts of food to lower the calorie intake. This results in failed diets in 95 per cent of cases. Successful dieting – to lose fat not protein – involves reducing carbohydrate intake in the form of 'bad' carbohydrates, to literally switch on our intrinsic fat-burning mechanism.

Vitamins and minerals

The simplest way of explaining vitamins and minerals is that they are substances that we require in small quantities in our diet. Absolutely essential for well-being, they *must* feature in a healthy, weight-loss diet. Happily, they will be included naturally if you select the correct balance of foods. Vitamins and minerals are necessary to facilitate certain chemical reactions in our cells, and some (such as vitamins A, C and E and the mineral selenium) also function as antioxidants, which help to prevent diseases and ageing by mopping up what are known as 'free radicals'. But what exactly are antioxidants and free radicals?

In each individual cell in your body (of which you have trillions) there are thousands of chemical reactions occurring every second. To release the energy from food, these chemical reactions produce 'free radicals', which are essentially molecules that have lost an electron.

Free radical formation

Molecule   →   losing electron   →   Free radical

Their natural reaction is to try to take an electron from another molecule, which will cause damage to the cells in your body – especially as this is occurring millions of times per second.

Free radical →   Free radical 'steals'   →   New free radical
                electron from another   formed
                molecule

This is not good, as it sets off chain reactions of 'stealing' electrons, which weaken your cellular defences against disease and infection. Obviously, you need to stop the process by 'wiping up' the free radicals before they can cause any damage.

This is where antioxidants come into the picture, our knights in shining armour! Antioxidants mop up the free radicals, preventing damage (and long-term disease), keeping us healthy, and delaying the ageing process. They are the closest we have come to the elixir of life in over one million years of existence.

Where do these wondrous things come from? Antioxidants occur in two main forms: as naturally occurring proteins in the body (which we make from essential proteins in our diet), and as various constituents in our diet that are necessary for the proteins to do their job effectively. These 'various constituents' are essential fatty acids (from eggs, oily fish and certain vegetable oils), and vitamins and minerals (from beef, pork, lamb, poultry, fish, shellfish, fresh fruit and vegetables, and dairy produce).

All of the essential vitamins and minerals we need are supplied in dairy produce, fresh vegetables, and animal foods (beef, pork, lamb, fish, poultry, eggs). And as several of the vitamins are *fat soluble* (vitamins A, D, E and K), we need a certain amount of fat in the diet for their effective absorption.

Now where have you seen this particular list of foods before?

The rest of Part I will provide guidelines for implementing the principles of the diet (and Part II features lots of delicious recipes that will enable you to put the diet into practice), but now you can see that if you eat the correct foods, in the correct proportions, you will lose fat naturally and without hunger, become much healthier, and at the same time increase your protection against disease and ageing. And all this will cost little or no more than you spend on food at the moment, and take no more time out of your day. Now you will begin to appreciate that what seemed too good to be true at the start of the book actually makes sense. And for the first time on any diet you understand what you are doing, and you are in control.

Chapter 5

The Golden Rules for a Successful Diet

Now that you understand the basis of this new system of eating (and therefore dieting), you can begin the process of removing excess fat forever. The beauty of this system is that your body's hormones do the work for you. In other words, your body will automatically reduce your weight to the level that is right for you, at the safest healthy rate for the human body, then automatically stop. You are not artificially manipulating your body (as on other diets), you are simply allowing your body's hormones to remove excess body fat medically. Obviously, you must have a realistic body image – waif-like proportions are not normal – but neither is the fat created by a modern diet of refined carbohydrates. You will lose weight easily by simply following the rules. Conversely, you won't lose too much weight on this diet. You are consuming high-quality protein and essential fats, vitamins and minerals, and when you reach your correct body weight, your hormones simply switch off the weight loss process; it seems too good to be true but it isn't. You provide the correct ingredients, as healthy food, and nature does the rest.

However, before commencing any diet you should discuss the matter with your GP, to ensure that there are no medical problems which make dieting unsafe for you. There are obvious situations, like pregnancy, where dieting is definitely contraindicated, but there are also many other conditions in this dieting may not be safe, and which may not be obvious to you. So always obtain your doctor's advice before dieting – or exercising.

As mentioned in a previous chapter, the diet consists of two parts: a weight loss phase and a weight maintenance phase. In the weight loss phase, you must restrict carbohydrates to less than 60 grams per day (and preferably less than 40 grams per day) to lose weight. When you are satisfied with your size (and try to base your decision on *size* not *weight*), or when the weight loss stops (which is your body's way of saying that this is your correct size), go on to the weight maintenance phase of the diet. I have emphasized *size* rather than *weight* because you are losing fat on this diet (which, of course, is exactly what you want), but fat is much lighter than protein, so you will reduce in *size* more than you reduce in *weight*. In fact, weight is a dreadful way of measuring the success of a diet, because, generally, the more weight you lose, the more body protein you lose, which is very dangerous.

As this system is really a way of life rather than a diet, you will find by the weight maintenance stage that you no longer crave refined carbohydrates, and it should be reasonably easy to keep your weight stable, even though you are consuming more (but not too much more) than 60 grams of carbohydrate per day. If you find your weight creeping back up, cut down the carbohydrates and it will soon reduce.

How to cut down on carbohydrates

As you will have appreciated by now, this medically based diet works by switching on the fat-burning mechanism we each have as an intrinsic part of our body chemistry. If you switch off the fat-storage mechanism, and switch on the fat-burning mechanism, you will lose fat. This depends entirely upon severely restricting your carbohydrate intake, especially in the early stages of the diet, because it is primarily carbohydrates (not fat or proteins) that stimulate insulin production – the hormone that promotes fat storage. So there is no possibility of 'cheating', even a little, on this diet. If you include the occasional cake or chocolate or pasta, the diet will not work.

So, the number one rule of the diet is as follows:

Eat no more than 40–60 grams of carbohydrate a day

Ideally you should try to keep below 40 grams of carbohydrate per day, and certainly below 60 grams. A single slice of bread alone is 17 grams of carbohydrate, so you can see that the carbohydrate limit is very strict. Of course, no-one is perfect and you are bound to break the rules occasionally, but you *must* try to keep to less than an absolute maximum of 60 grams of carbohydrate per day. If you exceed this level, the insulin response is almost certainly going to be activated, and suddenly all of the unlimited amounts of high-protein foods in your diet will be deposited as fat, and the fat-burning mechanism is switched off.

In practice, this means no breakfast cereals, milk (though cheese is allowed), cakes, biscuits, pies, potato crisps, potato chips, or most refined pre-packaged foods – and virtually no bread. It also means no refined sugar of any nature. And definitely no potatoes, pasta or rice.

These foods are very high in carbohydrate content, and must be avoided completely in the weight-loss stage of the diet. Later, you can re-introduce limited amounts of wholemeal bread, wholemeal pasta and wholemeal rice, which are rich in vitamins (such as thiamin) and fibre. Wholemeal products slow the digestive process, helping to prevent the massive fluctuations in blood sugar levels which are characteristic of the absorption of foods made from white, refined flour. Potatoes have a high starch component, and although they are an excellent source of nutrition, they must be avoided initially to reduce the insulin response and promote fat loss.

But to keep to the 40-gram limit, you also have to be wary of some other foods, as follows:

Restrict fruit in the weight-loss stage of the diet

I dislike this rule, but unfortunately it is necessary at first. All fruit is good for you. It is full of vitamins, minerals and fibre, and has a very high antioxidant capacity. Unfortunately for the dieter, many fruits also have a high sugar content. Now, these sugars are *natural* rather than *refined*, and are therefore much better for you than those found in cakes and sweets, but the insulin response cannot differentiate between one type of sugar and another, so you do have to limit severely the amount of fruit you eat in the weight-loss stage of the diet. If possible, omit fruit entirely from your diet, apart from an orange per day to maintain safe vitamin C levels. Of course, if you take a diet supplement tablet which contains your daily requirement of vitamin C, you could replace the orange with another piece of fruit, such as an apple or a peach. Check the table on page 270 to find out the carbohydrate content of various fruits. In general, most pieces of fruit contain 10–15 grams of carbohydrate each, so be careful. Bananas, however, are definitely out. As soon as you proceed to the weight-maintenance stage of the diet, re-introduce fruit at the earliest possible opportunity.

Vitamin C is essential for good health and has many important actions, not least its wonderful antioxidant properties. It is one of the few nutrients that we cannot obtain from animal foods (apart from liver). Although many vegetables are excellent sources of the vitamin, citrus fruits are the simplest way of preventing deficiency; a single orange provides your daily requirement of vitamin C – hence the one-orange-a-day allowance during the weight-loss phase of this diet. You will notice that many of the suggested recipes incorporate fresh lemon or lime juice, both for flavour and nutrition. However, even a single orange contains about 15 grams of carbohydrate (about the same as one slice of bread), and you have to keep your daily carbohydrate intake to less than 40 grams per day, if possible, to continue the fat-burning mechanism. So if you can replace the orange (or lemon) with a vitamin C supplement in tablet form, you will significantly reduce your daily carbohydrate intake.

No fruit juices

Fruit juices are high in sugar content (even the 'unsweetened' variety) and are totally excluded from this diet. This includes *all* fruit juices, commercial and freshly squeezed; they may have different sugar contents, but they all have too much sugar for a low-carbohydrate diet. You will obtain all the vitamins, minerals and antioxidants you need from other components of this diet.

Cut out virtually all milk – even skimmed milk

This restriction is so important that it is worth emphasising, as it is one of the commonest reasons for the failure of a low-carbohydrate diet; the sugar in milk is often forgotten. All milk, even low-fat skimmed varieties, has a high carbohydrate content (as lactose). So if you drink milk, you will exceed the acceptable carbohydrate intake. You can allow yourself perhaps a very little milk in tea, but no more.

The main value of milk is as a source of calcium and vitamins, which are easily provided by the cheese and other constituents in your diet. Cheese and cream are unrestricted because they are virtually carbohydrate-free, so they don't upset the diet. In effect, no carbohydrate, no problem.

No pulses or grains in the weight-loss stage of the diet

Once again, I dislike this restriction, because pulses and whole grains are rich in proteins, vitamins and minerals. Unfortunately, however, they also have a high carbohydrate content, so you'll need to cut them out to begin with. But as soon as the weight-loss phase of the diet is over, you can start cooking with them again.

Stick to low-calorie soft drinks

This particularly refers to carbonated fizzy drinks. This is not because regular soft drinks are high in calories but because they have a high sugar – and therefore a high carbohydrate – content. If you would like a soft drink, use the low-calorie equivalent to prevent sugar from creating an insulin response. But remember, some diet carbonated drinks contain caffeine, which also stimulates the insulin response, so drink them in moderation. Better still, drink water.

Cut out beer

Alcohol is not prohibited on this diet, but beer is definitely out. Beer has a relatively high sugar content (maltose), and will seriously compromise the diet. Wine and spirits have a much lower carbohydrate content (spirits have virtually none), so they can be tolerated in the diet. I know it seems strange, because alcohol is well known to contain lots of calories, but the calorie content is not important in itself on a low-carbohydrate diet. If the carbohydrate content is restricted, the insulin response will be blunted, and the calories in alcohol will not be deposited as fat.

I certainly do not intend to promote alcohol consumption, but I have to tell you the facts as they are, and on this basis a moderate amount of alcohol (as wine or spirits) will not cause weight gain on this diet. In fact, there is significant evidence to suggest that a glass of red wine per day is actually beneficial in preventing long-term heart disease; the protective effect is thought to result from the antioxidants in the red wine. And a 120ml glass of red wine contains less than 1 gram of carbohydrate. The carbohydrate content of various alcoholic beverages is shown on page 277. A word of warning though: always check the carbohydrate content of *mixer* drinks, which are usually much higher in carbohydrates than is alcohol alone. Low-calorie mixers are your best choice.

One other point to remember is that alcohol generally increases the appetite and affects self-control, so if you drink too much you may eat more than you need or blow your diet by giving in to a carbohydrate craving. In other words, alcohol is not necessarily bad for either you or your diet – if taken *in moderation*.

Drink tea, not coffee

Try to avoid coffee, or at least reduce your intake considerably, not just because of the effects of caffeine, but because *coffee stimulates insulin production.* In other words, coffee accelerates the effects of carbohydrates by magnifying the insulin response. And insulin promotes fat storage. So stop drinking coffee to help you lose weight – even though coffee, by itself, has no calorie content.

Fortunately, nature has provided us with a perfect substitute – tea. Unlike coffee, tea has no untoward effects on sugar metabolism, and so it does not upset our fat-losing programme. And tea has very high levels of antioxidants. It was always presumed that green tea was healthier than dark tea in this respect, but recent research has shown very little difference between the two types in terms of antioxidant levels. Drink tea – but with either very little milk (preferably none), or with cream, which has no carbohydrate content, rather than milk. Lemon in tea tastes great and is nutritionally excellent.

So those are the foods you need to avoid. But one word of advice: don't exclude carbohydrates completely from your diet. Have the equivalent of a slice of bread per day. There are also complex carbohydrates in the vegetables included in the diet. If you abstain from carbohydrates completely, you will notice a strange taste in your mouth. This is down to substances called ketones, which are the breakdown products of fats, and are a warning that you are reducing the carbohydrates a little too much. If you would rather not have a slice of bread, you can substitute another carbohydrate food for this, examples of which are shown in the table on pages 269–70.

And here's what you can eat . . .

Although carbohydrate foods are out, there are still
hundreds of delicious meals for you to enjoy, such as trout
with lemon hollandaise sauce, pepper steak, moussaka,
beef stroganoff, sweet and sour pork, lamb curry with red
pepper, roast beef . . . The potential variations with this diet
are literally endless, and I have included lots of ideas and
delicious recipes for putting the diet into practice in Part II
of the book.

Don't worry, within a very short period you won't miss
carbohydrates. Your body will automatically readjust to a
healthy diet (which is one with no refined carbohydrates)
and the addiction to sugars (because that's what it is) will
simply disappear. That is the reason why you have to give
up virtually all carbohydrates, because if you cheat then
your body doesn't have a chance to readjust.

Have as much protein as you like

There is no restriction on *fresh* beef, pork, lamb, poultry,
fish (including shellfish), eggs or cheese (except some of
the processed cheeses). I have emphasised that this applies
to fresh animal products only, to differentiate from pre-
packaged foods, which can contain large quantities of
hidden carbohydrates and sugars.

Manufactured foods such as sausages can vary
enormously in their carbohydrate content; some contain
high proportions of carbohydrates, whereas others (such as
Polish kabanas) have virtually no carbohydrate content at
all – so you should try to acquire the simple habit of
reading the carbohydrate content on the labels. 'Pure'
proteins (meat, poultry, fish, shellfish and eggs) have
virtually no carbohydrate content, so it's much easier to

base your diet on these foods. As well as being the basis of a successful weight-loss diet, they are also full of healthy nutrients and flavour.

This does not mean that you will gorge yourself on protein foods; your metabolism will not allow this. In fact, we only overindulge in carbohydrate foods – or, more specifically, combinations of carbohydrates and fats, which is where the problem arises. We do not overindulge in 'pure' fats; our metabolism tells us when to stop, because fats satisfy hunger. If carbohydrates did the same, there wouldn't be a problem.

Plants, of course, are an excellent source of protein (although usually not 'complete' proteins. The exception is soya (and its derivatives), which is certainly a complete protein.

Don't worry about 'pure' fats

This is the strangest rule of all. You are on a diet, and not restricting fats! Well you *are* actually restricting fats, and particularly the 'bad' fats in your diet, by severely restricting the carbohydrates, because the worst fats in your diet are combined with carbohydrates – which, of course, you have eliminated. Your body automatically adjusts to the new equilibrium, and you will not suddenly gorge on butter, cheese, cream and eggs. Your body knows when to stop, and, just in case this mechanism is faulty, you have switched off the fat-storage hormone so you will excrete any excess fat from your body and not store it as extra fat.

Before you become overly concerned about the fat in your diet (which we have changed from 'bad' fats to 'good' fats), perhaps I should mention that there is a considerable body of medical evidence supporting the hypothesis that simply lowering the amount of cholesterol you consume will not necessarily lower your blood cholesterol level. In other words, eating a low-fat diet does not equate to having a low blood cholesterol level. I know this seems like dietary heresy after all you have been told about how essential it is to adhere strictly to a low-fat diet for your future health, but as a clinician I have to present the facts, and the facts are that many highly respected medical journals have recently published scientific papers that strongly refute the concept of 'low dietary fat equals low cholesterol and better health'. In simple terms, all fats are definitely *not* bad for you.

One final point. In my opinion, eggs get a very bad press from certain dietary 'experts'. This is because egg yolks contain cholesterol. Now, let us remember that we need a certain amount of cholesterol for many essential body functions (hormone production, nervous system functioning – including the brain – and cell membrane formation, to name but a few), so all cholesterol is not bad. Major studies of healthy adults have shown that one egg a day does not increase the risk of heart disease and stroke, and that two eggs a day actually increase the amount of 'good' cholesterol in your blood, which is protective against heart disease. So eggs are not bad for us. And just think of all of the nutrition in an egg; it is a source of many essential amino acids, antioxidants, vitamins and minerals – and the proportion of the various nutrients in an egg are exactly in proportion to our nutritional requirements. How typical of nature to get it right, and of us to get it wrong! I am not suggesting that you overindulge in eggs, but an egg per day is not harmful, and has so many amazing health benefits that it is incredible that eggs have been criticised in the first place.

Feast on fresh vegetables

Fresh vegetables have so much goodness that it is difficult to know where to begin listing the benefits. They provide vitamins and minerals in abundance, and therefore many of the essential antioxidants we need to protect against disease and infection.

Basically, you can include virtually all vegetables in your diet, apart from those high in starch, such as potatoes, parsnips, corn and pulses (peas, beans and lentils) – see Appendix 3 for a detailed list. The list of vegetables included in the diet far outweighs those excluded.

It is essential that you don't ruin the nutrition contained in vegetables by inappropriate cooking. Vitamins and minerals are lost from vegetables when they are chopped up too early, so prepare them just before you intend to cook them. Of course, this isn't always practical, in which case a sealed packet of pre-chopped fresh vegetables (which retain a significant amount of goodness) is an acceptable substitute. Nutrients also leach out when you boil vegetables in water, so try to steam them, cook them in just a small amount of water, or, better still, use a wok, as this method of cooking retains a lot of the inherent goodness in foods (for more on wok cooking, sees pages 69–70).

So there you have the rules of the diet. What could be simpler? If you are in any doubt as to which foods you can eat and which are best avoided, you will find several charts in the book. A list of 'forbidden' foods is shown on pages 58–59, and these should be avoided at all times during the weight-loss stage of the diet. In the maintenance stage, you can have some of the 'forbidden foods', in moderation, but remember, your body will have readjusted and you will no longer have carbohydrate cravings. The list is not all-inclusive, as sugars and other carbohydrates can be 'hidden', so read the label on any pre-packaged or processed food to check the carbohydrate content.

To help you stick to the 40-gram carbohydrate limit, lists of the typical carbohydrate content of common foods are shown on pages 58–60; the first list details foods with a low carbohydrate content which can be included in the diet, and the second details those with a high carbohydrate content which should be excluded. For example, if you have a 100-gram slice of chocolate cake (carbohydrate content 55 grams) or a 100-gram bar of milk chocolate (carbohydrate content 61 grams), you have already exceeded your carbohydrate allowance for the day. But if you have an apple (13 grams carbohydrate), a peach (9 grams carbohydrate) or a shortbread biscuit (11 grams carbohydrate), you'll be within the allowance. The recipes in Part II of the book will help you to create delicious meals within the daily 40-gram carbohydrate limit; you'll see that the carbohydrate content of each dish is indicated at the end of each recipe.

It's actually easier to *stop* eating refined carbohydrates completely (as you lose the taste for them) than to cut down your carbohydrate intake, but if you can't stop, use the tables on pages 269–77 for guidance in keeping your daily intake below 40 grams. If you follow the general guidelines of the diet, you won't have to count carbohydrate content at all, and I can assure you that you will be receiving all the necessary ingredients for healthy nutrition, too. Indeed, you will be eating highly nutritious natural food, and be slimming at the fastest *safe* rate for your body – the perfect combination for the serious slimmer!

The weight-maintenance phase

There is no 'after the diet', there is only 'after the weight loss'. This is a way of life, not just a new fad diet to lose body fat. If you adhere to the rules, you will lose fat, you will probably be eating a healthier diet than ever before, and you will find you no longer need your sugar fix. As I mentioned earlier, there is no definite carbohydrate limit at this stage of the diet, because everyone has a different tolerance for carbohydrates. You can gradually re-introduce fruit, root vegetables, pulses and milk, and, providing your weight doesn't increase, you're quite safe. Obviously, even the 'forbidden' foods (like cakes and pastries) can be reintroduced *in moderation,* but, as previously mentioned, you'll find that you don't *need* them as you did before, and you'll probably not over-indulge.

So the end of the weight-loss phase is signalled either by your satisfaction that you have lost sufficient weight (and you definitely will lose weight on this diet, unlike others), or when the weight loss stops, which is the body telling you to stop trying to lose weight. Once you are satisfied with your weight and shape (and *please* be realistic about your aims), you can reintroduce certain foods, which you had to restrict during the weight-loss phase because of their carbohydrate content but which are nevertheless excellent sources of nutrition:

- *Fresh fruit.* All fresh fruit is full of vitamins and minerals, and therefore high in antioxidants. Fruit can be re-introduced in moderation (preferably no more than two standard pieces per day) when you are satisfied with your weight.

- *Whole grains.* These foods are high in B vitamins (thiamin, riboflavin and niacin), vitamin A and vitamin E.

- *Full-cream milk and milk products.* Milk is like eggs: it naturally contains all the nutrients you need and in the correct proportions for health. It is well known to be an excellent source of calcium and vitamin D (for strong bones), but it also provides vitamins A, B_2, B_6 and B_{12}.

  Why do I always suggest full-cream milk instead of low-fat milk? Surely low-fat skimmed milk is healthier, with the same calcium content but lower fat content? Unfortunately, the mechanics of the body are not that simple; it *needs* fat to absorb both calcium and vitamin D, so if you drink low-fat milk, you actually absorb less than 10 per cent of the calcium, which rather tends to defeat the purpose of drinking milk! Use full-cream milk and you *will* absorb the necessary calcium and vitamin D.

- *Pulses.* Beans, peas and lentils are excellent sources of proteins. Although they are not 'complete' proteins (like animal proteins) they are easily elevated to 'complete' status by combining them with either whole grains or milk.

All of the nutrition contained in these temporarily excluded food groups is provided by alternative foods in the diet, so you will not be missing any of the necessary proteins, vitamins and minerals during the weight-loss stage of the diet. Fruit, milk, whole grains and pulses are very good sources of nutrition which are only being restricted for a short time to allow you to lose your unwanted body fat.

In fact, the only foods that you should severely restrict forever are those consisting mainly of refined carbohydrates, our old 'friends' the cakes, pies, pastries, commercial pizza (you can make a healthy one at home), crisps, chips (once again, you can make oven-cooked chipped potatoes at home) and most commercial 'fast' foods – but home-made burgers can be among the most nutritious of foods. And the word is *restrict* not *omit*: you can have some foods with refined carbohydrates in your daily diet after you have lost weight – just reduce them to a low level of consumption and you should be fine. Your body will soon tell you if you're eating too much, because you'll put on weight.

A nutritionally safe diet

A responsible diet should allow you to lose weight easily and eat healthily at the same time. This diet does just that. You may be cutting out refined carbohydrates, but you will be receiving all the nutrients you need for your well-being from other food sources, as follows:

- *Essential amino acids.* These are provided by the proteins in animal products: meat, fish poultry, shellfish, eggs and dairy produce. While plants certainly have proteins, the only plant source with *complete* proteins is soya (and its derivatives). By contrast, all animal products have complete proteins (see page 29), so the easiest way to ensure you have all the amino acids you need is to eat meat, fish or dairy products.

- **Omega-3 fatty acids.** Most prevalent in oily fish such as salmon, mackerel, herrings, sardines and tuna, omega-3 fatty acids can also be obtained from egg yolks, as well as nuts and certain seeds (e.g. flaxseed oil).

- **Omega-6 fatty acids.** These are most prevalent in egg yolks, seeds (particularly sunflower, safflower and sesame), whole grains and some vegetables.

- **Vitamin A.** Typical foods with high concentrations of vitamin A are fish, egg yolk, butter, cheese, carrots, red peppers, spinach, tomatoes, and mangetout. This vitamin is present in most fruits and vegetables, but in varying proportions.

- **Vitamin B₁ (thiamin).** Excellent sources in this diet are pork, fresh fish (especially salmon), certain nuts (cashews, brazils, peanuts, pine nuts) and sesame seeds.

- **Vitamin B₂ (riboflavin).** This is present in dairy products (cream and cheese), liver, beef, chicken, eggs, fish, shellfish, mushrooms, avocado and almonds.

- **Vitamin B₃ (niacin).** High concentrations are found in fish (especially salmon and tuna), meat, chicken, liver and eggs.

- *Vitamin B$_6$ (pyridoxine).* This is present in fish (especially tuna), meat (particularly pork), liver, chicken, avocados, nuts (especially walnuts and cashews), tomatoes and tomato purée.

- *Vitamin B$_{12}$ (cyanocobalamin).* This is the only vitamin *not* found in foods of plant origin. It is present in highest concentrations in liver, seafood, fish (especially sardines, salmon and tuna) and eggs, and in lesser amounts in milk products and meats. Vegetarians are therefore recommended to take a vitamin supplement.

- *Folate.* The highest concentration of folate occurs in liver, but there are also good concentrations in most vegetables (especially green vegetables), meat, poultry, fish, shellfish, eggs and nuts (particularly peanuts and cashews).

- *Vitamin C.* Apart from liver and kidney, vitamin C is not present in animal products and has to be obtained from vegetables (especially red and green peppers, mangetout, tomato, and broccoli) and fruit (strawberries and citrus fruits).

- *Vitamin D.* This is where oily fish are in a class of their own, providing by far the highest levels of vitamin D compared with any other food group; mackerel, herring, salmon and, to a much lesser degree, tuna are particularly rich. There is a small amount of vitamin D in eggs and butter.

- *Vitamin E.* The dietary requirements for this vitamin are provided in the diet by nuts (almonds, hazelnuts, peanuts), olives, tomato purée, avocado and fish.

- *Vitamin K.* The best dietary source is undoubtedly green vegetables, such as broccoli, cabbage, lettuce, spring onions and spinach.

- *Selenium.* This mineral is vital for the production of enzymes, and is available in onions, tomatoes, broccoli, bean sprouts and fish.

- *Iron.* You will obtain sufficient amounts of this important mineral from fish, nuts, liver, meat, chicken, sesame seeds and green vegetables.

- *Manganese.* This is found in eggs, nuts and green vegetables.

- *Copper.* Nuts, mushrooms and green vegetables are all good sources of copper.

- *Zinc.* Excellent sources include eggs, sesame seeds, nuts (especially cashew nuts and almonds), herbs and many vegetables.

- *Potassium.* This is abundant in fish, herbs, garlic, onion, vegetables, mushrooms and citrus fruit.

- *Calcium.* Important for the manufacture of bones, this is found in dairy products, fish, green vegetables (especially broccoli and parsley) and herbs.

- *Sulphur.* You can obtain this from garlic, onions, fish, eggs, nuts, cabbage and meat.

Don't worry, you don't need to learn any of the details in the above list of nutrients. I have merely included it to show you, in a very simplistic way, that you are receiving all that you require for good health by following this diet, which allows unrestricted consumption of these essential nutrients, in the form of delicious meals. The recipes in Part II have been carefully devised to help you receive a nutritionally balanced diet; for more ideas on how to balance your meals, turn to the menu plans on pages 73–76.

What happens if you break your diet occasionally?

Unfortunately, this diet is not as forgiving as some others. In a calorie-control diet, you can eat some chocolate cake and make up for the extra calories by eating very little for the rest of the day – but low-calorie diets mess up the body's chemical balance and don't work.

In the low-carbohydrate diet, if you consume more than 60 grams of carbohydrate per day, your body will respond by depositing the excess calories as fat. So you can't have many lapses, or it simply won't work. A biscuit here and a pastry there and it will all go to fat. Of course, nobody's perfect (certainly not me!), and no-one can rigidly adhere to all the rules all the time. The occasional lapse with a sandwich or a piece of fruit will merely cause the diet to fail on that day only, but really this diet is so liberal that lapses will be infrequent. So don't panic if you break your diet occasionally, it's only human. By satisfying your natural hunger in a natural way, for the first time you have a diet that is working *with* you, not *against* you. Remember, within a few days of commencing the diet your body will automatically readjust, and you will no longer need sugars; the addiction will disappear. Your body will be on automatic pilot! And you will not be hungry during the early phase of the diet, the most difficult period in most diets.

And now to the good part!

After a few weeks on the diet, your body automatically adjusts to the new insulin levels. This means that you will almost certainly be able to eat more than 60 grams of carbohydrate per day after the weight-loss phase of the diet *and still not gain weight*. Obviously you can't eat too much or your weight will increase, but you will be able to 'mini-binge' safely on occasions.

This diet works – and it lasts!

Foods excluded from the diet

You'll need to cut out most carbohydrates, to ensure a daily carbohydrate intake of less than 40 grams per day. To avoid the hassle of carbohydrate-counting, which is almost as bad as calorie-counting, this essentially involves excluding the following foods:

- Bread – a maximum of 1 slice (preferably wholemeal) per day.
- Pasta
- Rice
- Flour
- Potatoes and certain other starchy vegetables (see pages 275–76)

- Refined sugar of any nature, especially cakes, biscuits, pastries, pies and processed or pre-packaged foods with 'hidden' sugars or carbohydrate content. Read the labels on food to determine how much sugar or carbohydrate is in it. Remember, most 'low-fat' foods are high in carbohydrates, so they are not good in this diet
- Breakfast cereals
- Milk (you can have a *very* little in tea, if necessary, but be careful not to ruin your diet with too much). Substitute cream or lemon if possible
- Yoghurt
- Coffee (if possible). If you can't exclude coffee, drink only decaffeinated coffee. Caffeine stimulates insulin production *without* sugar, so it is definitely not good for this diet
- Beer – far too high in sugar
- Fruits (except an orange or lemon per day) and in the first stage of the diet only. Fruit is re-introduced as quickly as possible when weight loss is proceeding at a satisfactory pace
- Fruit juice – commercial or freshly-squeezed
- Dried fruit
- Pulses (peas, beans, lentils) or grains, in the first stage of the diet. You can re-introduce these in the weight-maintenance phase, when you are satisfied with your weight

Foods included in the diet without restriction on quantity

- All fresh protein from an animal source: beef, poultry, pork, lamb, offal (such as liver), fish and

shellfish. Tinned tuna, sardines and salmon are also
unrestricted

- 'Pure' fats, such as butter, cream, olive oil (especially
extra-virgin olive oil), fish oils, nut oils and
mayonnaise (without added sugar)
- Eggs (preferably free-range)
- Cheese – all varieties
- Fresh vegetables, except those high in starch, such
as potatoes. You will find a list of vegetables you
can eat at any stage of the diet on pages 275–76,
and a list of vegetables you should restrict during
the weight-loss phase (primarily root vegetables) on
page 276
- Onions, which deserve a special mention, for their
high vitamin and mineral content, and excellent
antioxidant capacity
- Herbs, especially garlic and ginger
- Spices
- Low-calorie soft drinks (except those restricted by
their phenylalanine or caffeine content)
- Tea – an excellent source of protective antioxidants
- Artificial sweeteners – providing they do not
incorporate carbohydrates (most don't)

Chapter 6

The Diet in Practice

The beauty of this diet is that you don't have to count calories or settle for small portions. It is also a much easier way of losing weight than standard diets: you eat as much as you like of some foods, restrict carbohydrates, and you lose fat without really trying!

But it will involve a change in the way you think about food. For example, most of us are conditioned to consider carbohydrates as our primary 'fast' food, from cereals and toast with marmalade for breakfast, to pastries or biscuits at mid-morning, sandwiches or fried food at lunchtime, and pasta, rice or potatoes as a standard addition to the evening meal.

The typical carbohydrate-based diet

Breakfast	Mid-morning Snack	Lunch	Dinner
cereal	pastries	sandwiches	pasta
toast	biscuits	pasta	pizza
croissants		take-away:	curry
marmalade		pies	fish and chips
		Chinese	meat and
		Indian	potatoes
		burgers	take-away:
		pizza	(same as lunch)
		fish and chips	

These carbohydrates are self-serving: the more you eat, the more they stimulate insulin which rapidly lowers your blood sugar levels; this in turn makes you crave yet more sugar, which is then deposited as fat. So you need to stop thinking of carbohydrates as the 'main event' of your meals, and base your diet instead on meat, fish, poultry and vegetables. Bread, rice, pasta and potatoes are merely the 'support act'; they provide bulk to your diet – and more energy than you require, which is stored as excess fat. You don't need them, and should therefore exclude them from your diet – at least while you are in the process of losing fat.

Have a substantial breakfast

How many times have you heard that breakfast is the most important meal of the day? This is true, but it's also true that you have to eat the right kind of breakfast, especially if you are trying to lose fat. There is no point filling up on carbohydrates at breakfast – bread, jam, marmalade, cereal, milk and sugar – because they only stimulate an insulin response, your blood sugar drops within 1–2 hours, you become hungry and slightly irritable, and eat more carbohydrates (such as biscuits, pastries or cakes) to compensate. And thus the vicious circle continues.

So when you are actively losing weight, you should stick to an absolute maximum of one slice of bread (or equivalent) per day, and avoid all cereal, grains and sweet food (except fruit, and even that has to be severely restricted during the weight-loss phase) for breakfast. In addition, try to cut out virtually all milk, as it is relatively high in sugar; a little milk in tea or coffee is all that is allowed, and even that should be replaced by cream if possible.

Don't worry, you won't starve without bread and cereals for breakfast; in fact, you won't even be hungry. These will be replaced by eggs (fried, boiled, poached, omelette, scrambled), bacon, gammon, cheese, mayonnaise, mushrooms, chicken, ham, fish (especially smoked) . . . The possibilities are endless! You'll find dozens of mouth-watering breakfast recipes in Part II.

The other reason that you should eat a substantial breakfast low in carbohydrate but with some fat content is because fats satisfy your hunger and slow the absorption of food from the intestines. In other words, you will be satisfied after the meal and won't feel hungry for hours – which is exactly what you are trying to achieve.

The only problem is time. Most of us are in too much of a rush to prepare breakfast first thing in the morning. Or so we are indoctrinated to think! In fact, it takes no longer to cook boiled eggs, or scrambled eggs (very easy in a microwave), poached or fried eggs with toast and either bacon or grilled gammon than it does to eat polystyrene cereal and toast with marmalade. With a breakfast of eggs and bacon (or grilled gammon steak), not only do you start the day with a substantial meal that tastes good, but you also act in the best interests of your health by having a high-protein, low-carbohydrate meal. The protein, vitamins and minerals from the bacon/gammon and eggs cannot be bettered by synthetic foods, and the fat will *naturally* satisfy your hunger for hours by encouraging a slow, steady absorption of food from the bowel, rather than the rapid absorption, and rapid hypoglycaemia, that follows the ingestion of refined carbohydrates. And if you don't like eggs, you can still choose from fish, cold meats, poultry, cheeses . . . Hardly tasteless fare!

Fish may seem a strange thing to eat early in the morning, but kippers or poached fish were popular breakfast dishes until a few decades ago. They taste wonderful, take very little time to cook, and really set you up for the day – they have virtually no carbohydrate content, and contain natural fish oils which slow the absorption of food and are an excellent source of essential fatty acids and antioxidants.

For those who are really pressed for time in the morning, continental ham, sliced meats and poultry, cheese and hard-boiled eggs are marvellous. These need not be expensive. Just two to three slices each of pre-packed ham and cheese with a hard-boiled egg (which cooks itself while you are showering) make an excellent 'fast' breakfast that is also very nutritious and highly 'diet-conscious'.

A wide selection of healthy, nutritious, low-carbohydrate breakfasts is given in Chapter 7.

Light bites and working lunches

It is easy to incorporate lunch into the low-carbohydrate diet. There are several distinct categories of lunch to consider, as different people have different lifestyles: packed lunch, take-away lunch, restaurant lunch and lunch at home. The different approaches to each of these are explained in Chapter 8.

Main meals

More substantial lunches, or dinner, permit an almost infinite array of possibilities, from chicken and pepper frittata to salmon with lemon butter sauce or beef stroganoff. Meals are no longer based on starchy foods, like rice or pasta or potatoes, but rather on nutritious foods such as meat, fish, poultry and vegetables, with delicious sauces to complement the food. An extensive, but by no means comprehensive, list of possible recipes is contained in Part II.

You'll see that there are no desserts in this book. The main reason for this deliberate omission is that you have to break the body's addiction to carbohydrates. If you have dessert, even with low-carbohydrate artificial sweeteners, your body won't be able to readjust, and you won't break the addictive cycle. You have to avoid sweet foods to allow your body to readjust, which it will do in a relatively short period of time.

Safe snacks

Snacking between meals will be less of a problem on this diet than it is on others as your hunger will be naturally satisfied by the foods included in this diet – and it is hunger, not just bad habits, that causes you to snack. In other words, your previous diet failures were *not* your fault: you were simply hungry, and compensated by eating the wrong food. So it really is essential to have a substantial breakfast as this prepares the body for a successful dieting day.

If you must snack, choose judiciously, referring to the lists on pages 269–74 to keep within the 40–60-gram carbohydrate limit. But be careful, it's not worth ruining your diet for the sake of one or two snacks per day. If you are regularly peckish between meals, you probably need to eat more at mealtimes. Providing you stick to the carbohydrate limit, you will not gain weight even if the meals are larger.

There really aren't many safe snacks on a low-carbohydrate diet, because there aren't many snacks that consist of pure protein and fat. By far the best in this regard is nuts, virtually all varieties (except chestnuts and cashew nuts) are low in carbohydrates, have substantial amounts of protein, vitamins and minerals, and are very filling. But I can't emphasise enough that it really is better to eat larger meals to prevent the need for snacking.

Shopping: the secret of successful dieting

All the ingredients for this diet can be planned and purchased on just one shopping trip a week. Your aim is to ensure you always have the following foods to hand:

- *Herbs and spices – fresh and dried.* These not only taste good, but also have a very high concentration of antioxidants, which are essential in the promotion of good health. They do not deposit fat and are easily added to recipes to enhance the taste, so they improve both health and flavour at the same time – simply perfect!

  You'll use fresh herbs almost every day, so they won't be wasted. You could also consider growing the herbs yourself, either in your garden or in small pots in the kitchen, for instant availability. Keep a good supply of dried herbs and spices – such as cumin, coriander, turmeric, cinnamon, paprika and chilli – in your store cupboard, too. They can be a little expensive to buy initially, but they last a long time and will enhance countless meals

- *Garlic.* This is one of the most nutritious foods known, with high quantities of vitamins and minerals. It is also an excellent source of antioxidants. So unless you really dislike the taste, try to incorporate garlic in your cooking as often as practically possible. It has been shown to protect against heart disease, cancer and even the ageing process itself through its incredible antioxidant properties

- *Onions*
- *Fresh vegetables*, especially peppers (red, green and yellow, because they have different vitamin concentrations), carrots, broccoli and spring onions
- *Extra-virgin olive oil*
- *Fresh ginger root*. This is a particularly useful herb in many dishes and has marvellous health-giving properties
- *Cheese(s)*, according to taste
- *Sour cream*
- *Mayonnaise*
- *Free-range eggs* – large
- *Fresh beef, poultry, pork or lamb*, according to taste
- *Fresh fish*
- *Tinned tuna* (preferably in brine)
- *Frozen prawns*
- *Oranges and lemons*
- *Tomatoes*. Try to eat these as regularly as possible, as they contain a powerful antioxidant called lycopene, so stock up on both the fresh and tinned varieties. Plum tomatoes have the highest concentration of lycopene, and unusually this health-giving nutrient is actually more prevalent in *cooked* tomatoes than it is in raw ones
- *Black peppercorns*

Other foods that you will need occasionally include:

- *Shellfish*
- *Tomato purée*
- *Dijon mustard*
- *Tomato juice*
- *Nuts* – virtually any kind, according to personal preference: macadamia, almonds, brazils, walnuts, hazelnuts and occasionally cashew nuts (as these have a much higher carbohydrate content)
- *Limes*

Remember, these ingredients are replacing items you would normally buy, not in addition to your usual shopping bill, so the cost factor is not high. These foods will naturally re-programme your eating habits, so you will begin to require less food without the necessity for either effort or will-power on your part.

Additional recommendations for the diet

The wide variety of foods included without restriction means that this diet is very easy to follow: the guidelines are simple and because you won't feel hungry, you are less likely to deviate from it. You have a very wide latitude in the types of foods that can be included, and Part II provides delicious recipes which are the essence of the diet. Here are a few extra tips to help you adhere to the diet:

Vary your menu as much as possible

You will find the diet easier to stick to if you base your meals on as wide a range of ingredients as possible. Not only are you less likely to get bored (and therefore risk snacking on forbidden carbohydrate foods), but you will also reap greater health benefits. The recipes in Part II of the book have been specially devised to provide as varied a diet as possible. The vegetables have been deliberately selected for their nutritional content: for example, red peppers contain more than 20 times the vitamin C content of lettuce, and more than 15 times the vitamin A content of green peppers. You can follow the standard dietary advice of eating five portions of any furit or vegetables per day and still not achieve goot nutrition if the fruit and vegetables you choose are not nutritionally balanced. These recipes are specifically designed to ensure excellent nutrition, providing you vary your daily menu. The secret of this diet is that it's not a diet, it's a way of life; if you follow the simple guidelines, you will slim and be nutritionally healthier – with virtually no effort.

Buy a wok

I would strongly advise anyone who wishes to lose fat, or even anyone who just wants to improve his or her health, to buy a wok. Although originating in an ancient era, wok cooking is ideally suited to our modern fast-paced lifestyle, as it allows the rapid cooking of tasty and highly nutritious food. And the variety of meals and combinations of ingredients that can be cooked in this way are almost infinite. For some strange reason, wok cooking seems to be ignored in most slimming recipes, and yet it involves cooking for short periods in small amounts of fat – and incorporates 'essential' fats which are vital for health. Heat can destroy vitamins, but wok cooking provides intense heat for a relatively short time, 'searing' meat and vegetables and thereby preserving most of the natural goodness in the food.

By cooking in a wok, you finish with a relatively high *volume* but a relatively small *amount* of food, because it has been chopped finely to allow rapid cooking. For example, a carrot, two spring onions, 10–12 florets of broccoli, a red and yellow pepper, a clove of garlic, and two slices of ginger root would be sufficient to provide a very substantial and nutritious vegetable dish for two people. The preparation time is ten minutes, the cooking time is five minutes, and the cost is relatively little. I give this example only to show how quickly, easily and cheaply fresh vegetables can replace pre-packaged 'convenience', foods.

Incidentally, I have no problems with lightly fried food, but I do not ever use deep-fat frying. I don't consider this form of cooking either healthy or necessary in modern society. Whilst sautéing in butter or olive oil is healthy (there really is no medical evidence to the contrary), deep-fat frying can destroy the very nutrition we are aiming to preserve for health.

Get exercising

Regular exercise will complement your diet; not only will it improve your shape and body contour, it will also make you feel much better because regular (simple) exercise improves the blood flow to the tissues of the body, making us look and feel better. You don't need to spend a fortune on a gym membership, simple exercises you can do at home – without expensive equipment – will actually achieve a better result. To this end, I have included a simple programme of isometric exercises on pages 249–68. Isometric means that you can do the exercise in the comfort of your own home (in minutes), and achieve the same result as if you had been to the gym for hours. It needs no equipment and no expertise. It also involves no embarrassment. By investing just 10–12 minutes per day, four days per week, you will improve the muscle tone beneath the disappearing layer of fat, further enhancing the change in body shape which complements the weight-loss programme. If you also walk for 15 minutes three times per week you will improve your cardiovascular health, too. Of course, all exercise programmes *must* be sanctioned by your doctor before you start. For more on the benefits of exercise, and a simple exercise programme, turn to pages 237–68.

Measure shape before weight

I would encourage you to use the changes in your body shape on this diet as the main criterion of success, rather than the more conventional measurement of weight loss. You will certainly lose weight (as fat) relatively quickly, but of much more significance is the way your body shape improves. This form of dieting promotes a natural body shape, which is particularly enhanced by the isometric exercise programme. It will not cause the haggard look that accompanies most calorie-control diets, because you lose fat *without* loss of the underlying body protein. You will lose fat smoothly over the body, allowing time for skin elasticity to recover, and therefore without the unsightly folds of excess skin that can occur with crash dieting. So look at your body shape as the diet progresses and watch the way that your clothes fit better, as this is a more effective measure of the diet's success than just weight loss. This type of diet has much more to offer in terms of body shape and health than the 'normal' calorie-control diet.

Drink at least four large glasses of water per day

Constipation is not a significant problem on the diet, but it can become one if you do not maintain hydration. Drink *at least* four glasses of water per day – in addition to any other drinks acceptable on the diet – and you should have no problem.

Take a multivitamin supplement

It is *very* unlikely that you will experience vitamin or mineral deficiencies on this nutritious diet (unlike many other diets). However, as a matter of safety, I always advise individuals on any diet to take a multivitamin tablet every day to ensure good health. Providing the tablet includes the daily vitamin C requirement (and most do), you no longer need to have an orange or lemon per day, saving 15 grams of daily carbohydrate intake in the process.

So now you have the knowledge to change your shape (and life) for ever, and actually have more knowledge and understanding of nutrition and health than many so-called experts, it's time for you to begin your new dietary way of life and lose weight permanently. If you have any further doubts, proceed to the delicious selection of recipes in Part II and these will be dispelled immediately.

To demonstrate how easy it is to follow the New High Protein Diet, here is a possible 2-week starter plan, but these are just suggestions. As you have seen, the beauty of this diet lies in the immense variety of foods that are included *without restriction*. On this diet, you really will eat yourself thin, and enjoy the experience.

Monday

Breakfast: 2 scrambled eggs with Parma ham
             Single slice of buttered toast
Lunch: Smoked salmon and sour cream salad
Dinner: Beef casserole with chives
Total daily carbohydrate per person: 41 grams (24 grams without toast)

Tuesday

Breakfast: Baked haddock with grilled Swiss cheese
Lunch: Omelette with filling (tomatoes/mushrooms/herbs)
Dinner: Lamb skewers with cucumber raita
Total daily carbohydrate per person:15 grams

Wednesday

Breakfast: Fried bacon, mushrooms and tomato
Lunch: Tuna mayonnaise sandwich with herbs and red pepper
             Single slice of buttered bread
Dinner: Ginger scallops with mangetout
Total daily carbohydrate per person: 30 grams (13 grams without bread)

Thursday

Breakfast: Egg mayonnaise with tomato and basil
             Single slice of buttered toast
Lunch: Chicken drumsticks
             Tomato and avocado salad
Dinner: Sliced beef in oyster sauce
             Stir-fried vegetables
Total daily carbohydrate per person: 44 grams (27 grams without toast)

Friday

Breakfast: Continental breakfast
             (sliced cheeses, ham, chicken)
             Slice of buttered bread
Lunch: Tandoori chicken
             Crispy green salad
Dinner: Poached salmon with ginger

Total daily carbohydrate per person: 46 grams (29 grams without bread)

Saturday

Breakfast: 2 eggs (poached/fried/scrambled)
             Bacon and mushrooms
Lunch: Lemon sole with asparagus
Dinner: Roast duck with juniper berries and orange
             liqueur sauce
             Carrots, mangetout and yellow squash

Total daily carbohydrate per person: 23 grams

Sunday

Breakfast: Kipper(s): one or two
             Plum tomato and dill
Lunch: Roast beef
             Carrots, peas
Dinner: Piperade

Total daily carbohydrate per person: 20 grams

Monday

Breakfast: Gammon steak
             Tomatoes and mushrooms
Lunch: Avocado, tomato and Mozzarella sandwich
             (single slice of buttered bread)

Dinner: Swordfish steaks with lemon and garlic
Total daily carbohydrate per person: 36 grams (19 grams without bread)

Tuesday

Breakfast: 2 poached eggs with tomato
              Single slice of buttered toast
Lunch: Barbecued chicken wings (from supermarket
              or home)
              Feta salad
Dinner: Moussaka

Total carbohydrate content per person: 48 grams (31 grams without toast)

Wednesday

Breakfast: Lemon sole with herbs
Lunch: Turkey breast with gravy
              Asparagus
Dinner: Ratatouille

Total daily carbohydrate per person: 22 grams

Thursday

Breakfast: 2 boiled eggs
              Parma ham and plum tomato
Lunch: Prawn mayonnaise sandwich
              (single slice of bread)
Dinner: Pork chops with herbs
              French beans and carrots

Total carbohydrate per person: 28 grams (11 grams without bread)

Friday

Breakfast: Toasted cheese with chives and basil
             Single slice of buttered toast
Lunch: Cod with parsley sauce
             Baby leeks
Dinner: Grilled pepper steak with French beans

Total daily carbohydrate per person: 30 grams

Saturday

Breakfast: Eggs Benedict
             $^1/_2$ toasted muffin
Lunch: Mussels in tomato sauce with oregano
Dinner: Lamb's liver with mushrooms

Total daily carbohydrate per person: 45 grams (30 grams without muffin)

Sunday

Breakfast: Sliced ham and turkey
             Selection of cheeses: Edam, Gruyere, Chedder,
             Emmental
             $^1/_2$ toasted muffin
Lunch: Roast lamb
             Carrots and French beans
Dinner: Scallops and asparagus with sweet chilli sauce

Total daily carbohydrate per person: 30 grams (15 grams without muffin)

PART II

Recipes

Before I proceed with suggestions for meals which are both nutritious and slimming, there are a few simple principles to be outlined in the preparation and cooking of vegetables. You are probably already aware of these facts, but it's important to emphasise them as it's obviously essential to maintain as much of the nutrition and goodness in the vegetables and not lose the benefits by poor preparation and cooking techniques.

- Prepare vegetables as near the time of cooking as possible. Vegetables start to lose nutrients as soon as they are chopped, so try not to prepare vegetables in advance if possible. Obviously, however, we have to be practical. If you simply don't have time to prepare the vegetables yourself, use packs of chopped vegetables, which are readily available from supermarkets. These have lost some of the nutrients, but still provide a useful alternative in our hectic lifestyle, and are definitely better than reaching for the crisps or tin-opener.

- Lightly-steam, stir-fry or boil vegetables in as little water as possible, as this maintains the maximum nutrition.

- Never keep prepared vegetables covered with water. Nutrients leach out of vegetables quickly, and you can destroy their nutritional value by soaking them in water. Prepare vegetables at the last minute, and cook them as soon as possible.

- Add herbs and spices at every possible opportunity. Apart from the natural flavour enhancement, the nutritional benefit is immense. For example, paprika has over 10 times the vitamin A content of cabbage or green peppers, both of which are in themselves good sources of vitamin A.

- Eat the garnish! The purpose of garnish is to enhance the meal itself, not only its appearance. The garnishes utilized in these recipes are selected for both visual and nutritional content; don't leave them at the side of the plate.

- Vary the quantities in the recipes and still lose weight. The beauty of this diet is that the recipes are not cast in tablets of stone, unlike most other diets. If it is your preference to add more meat, or fish, or chicken, or vegetables, you can – without impairing the success of the diet in any way. Providing the additional ingredients are low in carbohydrate content, and you keep within your 40-gram carbohydrate limit, you can vary your menu according to taste without limits on quantities. What could be easier? All you have to do is to plan your shopping in advance, and your weight loss is assured.

- Fresh mayonnaise tastes better, but, once again, commercial products are effective and satisfactory substitutes for the real thing. Some commercial mayonnaise even includes a significant omega-3 fatty acid component. But remember always to check the label for any undesirable ingredients.

- Many of the recipes in this book include Lebanese cucumber, which has the advantage of a lower carbohydrate content than the English variety, but obviously any cucumber will suffice.

- The recipes are usually for two people; however, the quantities of ingredients can be varied proportionately if either more or less people are involved: double the quantities for four, or halve for one. Bear in mind that these recipes are not just *diet* recipes, they are *normal* high-quality meals (both nutritionally and gastronomically) which may be served on any social occasion. Your can entertain guests and provide them with a healthy weight-loss diet without their knowledge! How much more considerate could you be as a host/hostess? You are caring for your guests' health and longevity, as well as their social entertainment.

Chapter 7

Breakfast

Not many people consider having a cooked breakfast nowadays, mainly because it is considered too time-consuming. In actual fact, there is little additional time involved, and the nutritional benefits are immense. But there are still many alternatives.

Incidentally, you will notice in many of the breakfast dishes that fresh herbs are included, both for flavour and nutrition. But how are you to obtain fresh herbs every morning? Simply grow them yourself, either in the garden or in pots on the window-ledge. They are easy to grow, require little effort, cost very little to buy initially and are instantly available. The difference fresh herbs make to even the simplest of dishes is immeasurable and the cost factor insignificant.

In the following recipes you will see that I have very slightly broken some of my golden rules: occasionally you will see a little milk included in a recipe, or a teaspoon of sugar, or even a tablespoon of flour. These small quantities in a recipe for several people will make no difference to the overall carbohydrate content of the diet, and will improve the taste immensely.

Eggs

Eggs, in any form, are included to great effect, in terms of both healthy diet and gastronomic pleasure, in our breakfast menu. They are very high in protein, vitamins, minerals and antioxidants, with virtually no carbohydrate content, and the fat ensures a slow, even absorption of food. The potential variations on delicious recipes in which this versatile food can be used are almost limitless. Eggs will reappear in the supper section; however, in the breakfast menu I have concentrated on those dishes that can be prepared quickly.

Scrambled eggs

Scrambled eggs are probably better when cooked by the traditional method in a pan; however, this is definitely time-consuming, and may not be practical for everyone first thing in the morning. Fortunately, this dish can be quickly cooked by microwave for those who prefer. I will describe both methods and you can choose which is best for your own situation.

For 2

4 large eggs (preferably free-range)
2 tbsp full-cream milk
freshly ground black pepper
25 grams butter

Traditional method

Break the eggs into a mixing bowl, add the milk and a little freshly ground black pepper, and beat gently with a fork to an even consistency. Melt the butter in a small pan over a low heat and add the eggs. Stir constantly, moving the edges to the middle with a circular motion, for about 2–3 minutes. Remove from heat when the eggs are no longer runny (before the eggs have set) to allow the heat of the pan to gently finish the cooking, and serve.

By microwave

Add the beaten eggs to a microwave-safe bowl and place in the centre of the microwave oven. Set oven to high and cook for one minute. Remove the bowl from microwave, and stir the mixture, bringing the edges to the centre. Return to the microwave, cook on high for another minute and then stir again. Repeat the process for another minute, or until the mixture is no longer runny.

This is, of course, the very basic recipe for scrambled eggs, and the possibilities for spicing it up are almost endless. Here are a few of the high-protein 'diet' foods that you can add, and continue to lose weight:

- Parma ham, finely chopped
- Smoked salmon, finely chopped
- 50 grams of grated cheese: Emmental, Jarlsberg and Gruyere are marvellous in this recipe
- 1 tbsp of fresh herbs, chopped finely and added to the mixture. Parsley, chives, basil, dill and tarragon can be added very effectively, either as individual herbs, or combined with the ingredients above.
- Button mushrooms, sliced, then lightly fried in a little butter
- Plum tomatoes (two), seeded and diced
- Bacon rasher, diced finely and lightly fried in butter.

Carbohydrate content per serve: **2–3 grams, depending on added ingredients**

Eggs are one of the very few foods which I consider it is almost impossible to enjoy without bread (our forbidden carbohydrate); however, restrict yourself to one slice of buttered wholemeal toast (which equates to 17 grams of carbohydrate in itself). Of course, if you can survive without toast, you can 'spend' your daily carbohydrate quota on an alternative source of carbohydrate, either at breakfast or later in the day.

Omelette

For 2
4 large eggs (preferably free-range)
freshly ground black pepper
pinch of rock salt
2 tbsp full-cream milk
25 grams butter

Whisk the eggs, seasoning and milk with a fork to an even consistency. Melt the butter in an omelette pan (or small frying pan), tilting the pan to ensure an even coating of butter. When the butter is hot but not burning, add the egg mixture. Stir the mixture with the fork until the omelette sets, then stop stirring. Cook the omelette for about another minute, then, using a palette knife, gently lift one edge of the omelette, fold one half over the other and slide the omelette onto a plate.

Omelettes can be an ideal meal for breakfast, brunch, lunch, dinner, or supper, depending on the occasion and the time available for preparation. They can be as simple or as complicated as you wish. The fillings described for scrambled eggs (such as Parma ham, smoked salmon, cheeses, herbs, tomatoes, mushrooms and bacon) are equally suitable for omelettes.

Frittata, an Italian modification of the French omelette, takes a little longer to prepare as it involves cooking the eggs more thoroughly to produce a more solid end-product. As the typical frittata takes 15 minutes of slow cooking, it may not be suitable for weekday breakfast. However, it can, of course, be prepared the previous evening and provide the perfect 'instant' nutritious breakfast. As frittata takes longer to cook, I have included it in the lunch/dinner section (see pages 211–12).

Carbohydrate content per serve: 2–3 grams (depending on added ingredients)

Boiled eggs

For 2

2 large free-range eggs

Probably the only meal that is even faster than opening the cereal packet! Place 2 large eggs in warm water, bring to the boil, then reduce the heat to a gentle simmer. Excessive boiling will spoil the flavour and often causes the eggs to crack. The length of simmering depends on how you prefer your boiled eggs: with large eggs, between 3 minutes for soft-boiled to 8 minutes for hard-boiled.

In my opinion, boiled eggs are impossible to enjoy without toast, but again restrict yourself to one slice of buttered wholemeal toast per person. Or you can hard boil the eggs and enjoy them with some finely sliced Emmental or Jarlsberg cheese, perhaps with some slices of Parma ham or finely sliced turkey breast. These latter ingredients sound expensive, but they are not. If you buy some cheese and a packet of sliced ham or chicken breast from the delicatessan, a little each day is actually very inexpensive. The restriction of carbohydrate in this diet decreases appetite to a normal level and reduces cravings for large quantities of food. In that respect, the diet is self-sustaining.

Carbohydrate content per serve: **negligible (without toast); 17 grams (with toast)**

Poached eggs

For 2
2 large free-range eggs

Once again, the wonders of modern science allow us to poach eggs either by the traditional method or more rapidly by microwave, which, while it may not seem very trendy, is immensely beneficial to those hard-pressed for time in the morning.

Traditional method
Heat the water to boiling point in a shallow pan, then reduce the heat to a gentle simmer. Break each egg individually into a cup, and slide the eggs gently into the boiling water. Cook for approximately 3–4 minutes, removing the eggs from the water with a perforated spoon when the yolk is evenly coated with a white film and the

white has cooked. Serve on a slice of buttered wholemeal toast.

By microwave
Break each egg individually into the plastic cups specially designed for microwave poaching of eggs. Pierce the top of the yolks four to five times with a sharp knife, add a teaspoon of cold water and close the sealed top of the cup. Cook on medium (careful, on high it will explode!) for about 1–2 minutes (depending on the power of the microwave), then allow to stand for another minute before serving.

Carbohydrate content per serve: **negligible (without toast); 17 grams (with toast)**

Eggs Benedict

The classic recipe includes Canadian bacon; however, this version incorporates prosciutto for a lighter flavour. The lemon hollandaise sauce can be prepared the previous day.

For 2
2 large free-range eggs, poached
1 English muffin
50 grams prosciutto
hollandaise sauce (see page 131)
chopped fresh chives, to garnish

Prepare the hollandaise sauce according to the recipe on page 131 but use only 1 teaspoon of lemon juice. Halve the muffin and toast each half lightly. Lay the prosciutto on each half muffin. Poach the eggs, place the drained poached eggs on the ham and top with hollandaise sauce, garnished with chopped chives.

Carbohydrate content per serve: **15 grams (including muffin)**

Fried eggs

Strange though it may seem, you *can* eat fried eggs on this diet and continue to lose weight at a very substantial rate. The secret lies in the lack of carbohydrate. If you don't stimulate the body to make fat, you won't deposit fat, and eating fried eggs is the proof of this statement. Many people simply don't like eating fried food, and I'm certainly not advocating that you start eating fried food just because it's permitted, but there are, in my opinion, few more enjoyable breakfasts than bacon and eggs.

I prefer to fry eggs in extra-virgin olive oil, both for the taste and also because the oil is so healthy. Pour about 4 tbsp of extra-virgin olive oil into the (preferably non-stick) frying pan. Heat the oil until it is hot but not burning, and gently crack the eggs into the pan. Then cook them to taste, either sunny-side up, over-easy (turning the eggs), or simply by basting the hot oil over them with a spatula. Once again, the duration of cooking is a matter of personal preference, depending upon how well you like your eggs cooked.

When cooked to taste, remove the eggs with a perforated spatula and serve either alone or with a combination of grilled bacon, gammon, mushrooms, or tomatoes.

Carbohydrate content per serve: **negligible**

Fish

Fish is not a common breakfast dish today, but that is
merely a reflection of modern society. It was not so very
long ago that fish was one of the staple dishes on the
breakfast menu, and there is really no reason why it should
not continue to be. It is the original fast food, with the
difference that it is full of virtually every kind of goodness
you can imagine: protein, essential fatty acids, vitamins,
minerals, natural antioxidants and virtually no
carbohydrate. And the dishes can be as simple or as
complicated as time will allow. For breakfast I am going
to concentrate on dishes which are relatively quick and
simple to prepare. Some of the more time-consuming fish
recipes are described later, but of course the choice is
yours.

Pan-fried lemon sole

*This is one of life's simple pleasures, and it
could not be more delicious. In my opinion, it
is a suitable meal at any time of day.*

For 2

2 lemon sole fillets
60 grams butter
lemon wedges
1 tsp chopped fresh basil
2 tsp freshly squeezed lemon juice
freshly ground black pepper

Heat the butter in the pan and saute the lemon sole fillets,
for about 1–1½ minutes per side, turning carefully once
with a fish slice. Serve the fillets onto warm plates. Add the

basil to the butter in the pan, stir in the lemon juice, and heat gently for a few seconds. Pour the sauce over the fish, season to taste and serve with lemon wedges.

The fillets can be dusted with flour if you prefer; however, with careful cooking – and in particular the use of a fish slice – they will not break up, and flour really doesn't add anything to the flavour. The avoidance of any unnecessary carbohydrate in the diet is a definite advantage.

Cod or haddock can substitute for lemon sole, but the larger fillets take longer, and are not as suitable for rapid cooking at breakfast.

Carbohydrate content per serve: 1 gram

Baked haddock

If you need a dish that takes virtually no preparation time and provides you with a delicious, nutritious breakfast, this is for you.

For 2

2 haddock fillets
100 ml full-cream milk
1 tbsp chopped fresh chives
1 tbsp chopped fresh basil
freshly ground black pepper

Place the haddock fillet in an oven-safe dish and add the full-cream milk and the chopped fresh herbs. Cover with pierced aluminium foil, and cook at 190 degrees C (gas mark 4) for 20 minutes. Drain, season to taste and serve with a slice of hot buttered wholemeal toast.

Baked haddock with grilled Swiss cheese

For 2

2 haddock fillets

100 ml full-cream milk

1 tbsp chopped fresh chives

1 tbsp chopped fresh basil

50 grams grated Emmental cheese

freshly ground black pepper

If you have just a few extra moments to spare in the morning, this variation on the baked haddock recipe is delightful.

Prepare the baked haddock according to the recipe on page 90. Drain the haddock and place it on a slice of hot, buttered wholemeal toast. Grate some Emmental cheese over the haddock and place under a hot grill for 30–40 seconds.

The Emmental can be replaced by Gruyere, Jarlsberg or Edam (the latter are certainly *not* Swiss cheeses, but are equally suitable for this delicious recipe) according to your personal preference. I consider Cheddar cheese a little too overpowering for haddock.

Carbohydrate content per serve: **3 grams** *(20 grams including toast)*

Scrambled eggs and baked haddock

For 2

2 baked haddock fillets (see pages 90–91)

2 scrambled eggs (see pages 82–83)

2 tsp Dijon mustard

freshly ground black pepper

fresh coriander leaves, to garnish

Bake the haddock and prepare the scrambled eggs (either in a pan or microwave) as described on pages 82–83. While the eggs are still slightly fluid, drain and flake the haddock, and stir the mixture into the scrambled eggs. At this stage, two teaspoons of Dijon mustard stirred into the mixture will add zest, but it is entirely to taste. Cook the haddock and egg mixture for a short time, until the eggs have almost set, and spoon onto a warm plate. Season with freshly ground black pepper to taste, and garnish with fresh coriander.

Carbohydrate content per serve: 3 grams

Poached eggs and smoked haddock

For 2

2 small smoked haddock fillets

1 bay leaf

pinch of rock salt

2 large free-range eggs

freshly ground black pepper

2 slices buttered wholemeal toast (optional)

Place the smoked haddock fillets in a deep frying pan, add hot water to just cover the fillets, then add the bay leaf and a pinch of rock salt. Bring to the boil and reduce the heat to a gentle simmer for about 3–4 minutes. In a medium saucepan, poach the eggs to taste (see pages 86–87). Transfer the cooked haddock fillets carefully with a fish slice to separate warm plates and place a poached egg on each haddock fillet. Add some freshly ground black pepper, and serve with a slice of buttered wholemeal toast (optional).

Carbohydrate content per serve: **negligible (17 grams with toast)**

Kippers

Kippers are among the world's great dishes – on their own! Sauces and accompaniments to dishes are the prerogative of many great gastronomic nations, but the Europeans have wonderful foods with natural taste, either directly from the sea, or manufactured by some of the greatest cheese-makers in the world.

The North Sea provides us with natural foods full of natural flavour; however, some enterprising and brilliant innovators in gastronomic cuisine – many hundreds (and possibly thousands) of years before the word 'cuisine' was in current usage – managed actually to improve on the natural taste of the fish by smoking it in a way that has remained unchanged (because it probably cannot be improved).

*Kippers can be cooked in many ways, but
the two easiest – and quickest – are frying and
poaching. Both are almost equally rapid,
equally nutritious, and equally tasty. The only
difference is individual preference.*

Fried kipper

For 1

1 kipper
60 grams butter
1 plum tomato, diced
1 tbsp chopped fresh dill
freshly ground black pepper
1 slice buttered wholemeal toast (optional)

Heat the butter in a shallow frying pan, add the kipper and
cook for 2 minutes on each side. Season to taste, garnish
with chopped tomato and fresh dill, and serve with a slice
of buttered wholemeal toast. The toast may be omitted if
you wish to reduce your daily carbohydrates.

*Carbohydrate content per serve: 3 grams (20 grams with
toast)*

Poached (or jugged) kipper

For 1

1 kipper
1 plum tomato, diced
1 tbsp chopped fresh chives

freshly ground black pepper
lemon wedges
1 slice buttered wholemeal toast (optional)

Remove the head, then place the kipper in a jug filled with boiling water, cover and leave for 4–5 minutes. Drain, season to taste, garnish with tomato and chopped chives, and serve with lemon wedges and a slice of buttered wholemeal toast.

What could be simpler, more nutritious, or quicker? In less than a minute, you have prepared a delicious meal, packed with protein, essential fatty acids, antioxidants, vitamins and minerals, and with virtually no carbohydrates – apart from the 17 grams in the slice of wholemeal toast, which is not absolutely essential. And it took less time to prepare than a bowl of cereal!

Carbohydrate content per serve: **3 grams (20 grams with toast)**

Mushrooms

Mushrooms are a magnificent source of vitamin B, they taste wonderful, (either alone or with fresh herbs) and they are quick and simple to prepare and cook. So unless you actually dislike mushrooms, remember to include *fresh* mushrooms in your diet. Mushrooms are equally enjoyable for breakfast, lunch, supper or dinner – or even as a late-night snack.

Mushrooms on toast

Simple title, simple preparation, but a delicious, rapid, and nutritious breakfast.

The flavour (but not the nutritional value) can vary dramatically with the type of mushroom used. I will describe a simple recipe with button mushrooms, but I would advise you experiment with various types of mushrooms to discover which flavour you prefer; mushrooms – like fish and cheese – are very much a case of individual preference, but all are equally nutritious, so you simply can't get it wrong. Button mushrooms are particularly useful in dieting as they have the same vitamin content but lower carbohydrate content than other varieties of mushroom.

For 2

150 grams button mushrooms
50 grams butter
1 tbsp chopped chives
1 tbsp chopped basil
pinch of rock salt
pinch of paprika (optional)
freshly ground black pepper
2 slices buttered wholemeal toast

Clean the mushrooms by wiping them carefully, and remove the lower half-centimetre from the base of each stalk. Cut the button mushrooms in half lengthways. Heat the butter in a medium saucepan, and add the mushrooms. Cook for about 2 minutes, stirring frequently, then add the herbs, salt and paprika. Season to taste and cook for a further 2 minutes. Remove the mushroom and herb mixture with a perforated spoon and serve on warm plates with buttered wholemeal toast.

*Carbohydrate content per serve: **1 gram (18 grams with toast)***

For the cook in a hurry in the morning, an even easier – and just as tasty and nutritious – mushroom breakfast can be prepared as follows.

> *For 2*
> 2 large flat mushrooms
> 50 grams butter
> 2 plum tomatoes, diced
> 1 tbsp chopped fresh coriander
> pinch of rock salt
> freshly ground black pepper
> 2 slices buttered wholemeal toast

Dice a plum tomato, mix with a little freshly chopped coriander, cover and set aside.

Wipe the mushrooms and trim the base of the stalks. Heat the butter in a shallow frying pan, sauté the mushrooms for approximately 2–3 minutes per side (depending on thickness), turning once, and serve on a slice of buttered wholemeal toast. Top with the tomato and coriander mixture, and season with freshly ground black pepper. Simple, nutritious, delicious and slimming!

*Carbohydrate content per serve: **2 grams (19 grams with toast)***

Cheese

One of the nice things about using high-protein, low-carbohydrate foods is that they are so adaptable and yet they all taste delicious on their own: meat, poultry, fish, eggs and cheese – the original fast food.

Don't pigeon-hole cheese into a snack or dessert food. Apart from last thing at night (when there are definite medical reasons for not eating it), cheese is adaptable to every mealtime. Breakfast is no exception.

Toasted cheese

Toasted cheese for breakfast can be served alone or with delicious accompaniments which are relatively inexpensive (in the small quantities involved) and yet quick to prepare and serve.

For 2

2 slices buttered wholemeal bread

grated cheese (cheddar, Edam, Gouda, Emmental, Gruyere or Jarlsberg)

freshly ground black pepper

This meal is limited only by your preference in cheese, because the almost unlimited variety of cheeses can provide a different breakfast every day of the year.

Lightly toast one side of a slice of wholemeal bread, then remove from the grill. Add grated cheese to the non-toasted side and return to the grill until the cheese has melted. Cheddar cheeses are excellent for this purpose; however, for variety try Edam, Gouda, Emmental, Gruyere or Jarlsberg – or whichever cheese you prefer. Add some freshly ground black pepper, then serve alone or with a little pickle.

For variety, freshly grated cheese can be mixed with the following additional ingredients before toasting, to provide a truly delicious breakfast:

- Parma ham, finely diced
- plum tomato, diced
- $1/4$ red pepper, deseeded and diced
- spring onion, finely chopped
- 1 tbsp chopped fresh chives and basil
- $1/4$ green chilli, deseeded and finely chopped
- 1 tsp of Worcester sauce and 2 drops of Tabasco sauce
- finely diced smoked salmon and 1 tsp chopped dill

Heaven on toast!

Carbohydrate content per serve: **17–18 grams (including the toast)**

Continental breakfast

This is a term which covers a multitude of sins, but in this context it is taken to mean a cold platter, easily and quickly prepared to provide a nutritious meal with virtually no carbohydrate content, and therefore ideal for the serious slimmer. Cheeses; slices of cold ham, chicken or turkey; boiled eggs; an orange (but no other fruit at the early stage in the diet); and a slice of buttered wholemeal bread or toast (optional) are all included, but definitely no croissants, pastries, jams or marmalade.

Chapter 8

Lunch on the Run

Lunches may be simply divided into those that are made for us (take-aways and restaurant meals) and those we prepare ourselves (packed lunches and meals at home). The difference is important when we are dieting to lose fat. Let's look at the various categories separately and see how easy it is to apply the principles of a low-carbohydrate diet to each situation:

Take-away

In most cases the term 'fast food' is merely a synonym for 'high-carbohydrate food', which is disastrous for an effective diet. Avoid chips, burgers, pies, quiche, pasta, pitta, rice and any of the other obvious sources of unwanted carbohydrates. Shish kebabs can be included – providing you have very little bread or pitta. Pre-packed sandwiches are acceptable, but be careful: keep to the restriction of only one slice of bread per day and make sure the fillings comply with our carbohydrate restriction guidelines. You can have an unlimited amount of tuna mayonnaise or prawn mayonnaise on the sandwich, but only one slice of bread. Certainly no cakes or pastries – but then, you knew that already!

Remember the other forms of take-away which are less obvious: the supermarkets for example. These outlets provide many forms of take-away foods which are eminently suitable to be included in a low-carbohydrate diet:

- chicken drumsticks and chicken wings (plain and with sauces, such as barbecue, tikka and Chinese)
- gourmet ham
- Chinese chicken and breast fillets
- Calamari
- smoked salmon

The list is almost endless. Check the carbohydrate content of the various foods and you will see that many pre-prepared fast foods in supermarkets are actually low in carbohydrates and therefore 'diet-friendly'.

Restaurant meals

If you intend to eat at a restaurant, choose meat, fish, poultry or pork *without* sauces. At home you can prepare sauces very effectively without sugar (and with a lesser amount of flour), but restaurants may not do so, therefore sauces are best avoided, as hidden sugars and can completely ruin your carbohydrate restriction and thereby ruin your diet. Providing you didn't have eggs for breakfast, eggs (cooked any way you like) are fine, as is mayonnaise. Add salad, vegetables without sauces (obviously no potatoes) or herbs to the main course without restriction. On these minimal restrictions, the choice in restaurant menus is immense.

Packed lunches

Packed lunches can be exciting or simple, depending upon the time you have available for preparation, but need never be boring, even if you have limited preparation time. Good food needs little preparation because it has its own natural flavours: what could taste better than the plethora of cheeses available, meat, poultry, fish, seafood and vegetables.

Chicken drumsticks

Chicken for breakfast involves either slices of pre-packaged chicken breast (served with ham and cheese in a continental-style breakfast) or chicken prepared the previous evening. Whilst chicken breast is wonderful at any time, chicken drumsticks seem to have much more flavour the next day, and essentially arrive pre-packed with their own 'handles' for the perfect self-contained fast food! Ideal for breakfast or lunch.

For 2

6 chicken drumsticks (with skin)
25 grams butter, cubed
freshly ground black pepper

Place the drumsticks in a single layer in the base of a shallow oven-safe dish and top with the butter cubes. Cover with pierced aluminium foil and cook in the centre of a pre-heated oven at 180 degrees C (gas mark 4) for 35–40 minutes. Remove from the oven and set aside to cool.

Carbohydrate content per serve: **negligible**

Sandwiches

You can, of course, prepare your own sanwiches as part of a daily carbohydrate restriction diet. In other words, no more than *one* slice of wholemeal bread per day (in the early stages of the diet). This restriction can be increased to two slices per day later in the diet, but obviously if you decide on a sandwich for lunch, you can't have any toast for breakfast. The important principle of this diet is to restrict carbohydrates; break the rule – even once – and you're back to square one for that particular day. You can eat as much as you want of the unrestricted foods and still lose weight *only providing you keep your carbohydrate intake below 40–60 grams per day.* If you eat more carbohydrate, the insulin mechanism is stimulated and the other foods in your diet (fats and protein) are working *against* you – instead of *for* you – by being converted into body fat.

Fillings for a sandwich need not be restricted to the standard diet fare, which is usually some form of salad – without mayonnaise, or with French dressing (*sans* sugar). The only restriction in this diet is carbohydrate content, not calories. So ensure that you butter the bread (or use margarine if you prefer), both for the vitamins in butter and the slowing of the digestion provided by the lipid content of the butter. All of these sandwiches can be prepared either as closed sandwiches or – even better – as open sandwiches. Providing the fillings are low in carbohydrate, the possibilities are almost endless, but you have to restrict yourself to only one slice of wholemeal bread per day. Previously, you were told to restrict calories, but now you have to learn to think in the opposite way: you have to restrict carbohydrate content – so sandwich fillings are largely unrestricted, but the bread becomes the problem. A selection of wonderful fillings which are entirely commensurate with a successful slimming diet are:

Avocado

For 2

1 small ripe Hass avocado, halved, peeled, stoned and
  finely sliced

with

either diced plum tomato or sliced Mozzarella cheese or
  both

2 slices buttered wholemeal bread

1 tbsp extra-virgin olive oil

2 tsp balsamic vinegar

freshly ground black pepper

Arrange the sliced avocado on a slice of buttered
wholemeal bread. Top with either diced plum tomato or
sliced Mozzarella cheese (or both). Drizzle the extra-virgin
olive oil and balsamic vinegar over the filling and season
with freshly ground black pepper.

*Carbohydrate content per serve: 3 grams (20 grams with
bread)*

Chicken

*There are so many different ways to use
chicken in sandwiches that I can only briefly
scrape the surface of possibilities here, but a
few delicious ideas follow. On a practical
level, unless you have more available time
than most of us in the morning, it is easier to
cook the chicken the previous evening,*

although obviously chicken does taste better freshly cooked. If there is no time to cook the chicken the previous evening, you can substitute sliced turkey or chicken breast from either a delicatessan or even a supermarket. Remember, while we are trying to make these meals as tasty as possible, they have to be practical for the modern world, because if you can't adhere to the diet, it won't work – which is the basic fault of most diets!

• Chicken with mayonnaise and avocado

For 2

1 small chicken breast fillet
2 tbsp extra-virgin olive oil
1 tbsp mayonnaise
half a small ripe Hass avocado, finely sliced
2 slices buttered wholemeal bread
freshly ground black pepper

Sauté the chicken fillet in the olive oil for approximately 5 minutes on each side, turning once, until cooked. Set aside to cool, then slice finely. Mix with the mayonnaise and spoon on to a slice of buttered wholemeal bread. Arrange the avocado slices on the chicken and season with freshly ground black pepper.

Carbohydrate content per serve: 1 gram (18 grams with bread)

• Chicken with Swiss cheese

For 2

1 small chicken breast fillet

2 tbsp extra-virgin olive oil
2 slices buttered wholemeal bread
1 tbsp tomato salsa (see page 232)
50 grams grated Emmental cheese
freshly ground black pepper

Prepare the tomato salsa according to the recipe on page 232. This can obviously be done the day before.

Sauté the chicken, as described on page 106, chop into cubes and arrange on a slice of buttered wholemeal bread. Spoon the tomato salsa on the chicken and add some freshly ground black pepper. Top with grated cheese of your choice. (I prefer Emmental or Jarlsberg for this sandwich, but cheese is such an individual taste that virtually any will suffice – with the possible exception of cheddars, which I personally find too overpowering a flavour for chicken.)

This can be served cold, as either an open or closed sandwich, or the open sandwich can be modified by placing it under a hot grill until the cheese has melted, to provide a delicious hot open sandwich.

Carbohydrate content per serve: **4 grams (21 grams with bread)**

Tuna

Tuna has the marvellous advantage over most of its fast-but-nutritious food rivals that it is instantly available from a tin, and the tinned variety retains its nutritional value entirely – the quintessential pre-packed food

*(almost unique in this respect). The only
disadvantage with tuna is . . . there isn't any!
It's a perfect ingredient in any healthy diet –
whether you need to lose weight or not.*

For 2

200-gram tin of tuna (in brine or springwater), drained

1 tbsp mayonnaise

1 tbsp chopped fresh basil

1 tsp chopped fresh coriander

freshly ground black pepper

2 slices buttered wholemeal bread

1 vine-ripened tomato, diced (optional)

1/2 small red pepper, deseeded and sliced thinly
   (optional)

1 tsp chopped fresh chives

Flake the tuna and mix with the mayonnaise, chopped basil
and coriander, and freshly ground black pepper. Spoon the
mixture liberally on two slices of buttered wholemeal
bread. This is delicious alone, or add diced vine-ripened
tomato (and/or sliced red pepper with chopped fresh
chives) for extra flavour and nutrition.

*Carbohydrate content per serve: **2 grams (19 grams with
bread)***

Eggs

*Providing you have not had eggs for
breakfast, you can have eggs for lunch
(assuming you like eggs, of course), either as*

an omelette or as one of the myriad of possible
sandwiches, a selection of which are described
on pages 105–9.

Salad

If you prefer gourmet salad sandwiches for
lunch, rather than the usual wet lettuce and
tomato, try the following, and still lose weight:

- tomato and avocado salad (pages 222–23)
- Feta salad (pages 223–24)
- avocado and mint salad (page 224)
- rocket and olive salad (pages 225–26)
- courgette and sour cream salad (page 226)
- Mozzarella and avocado salad (pages 226–27)
- tomato and Parmesan salad (page 227)
- radish and basil salad (page 228)
- crispy green salad (pages 229–30)
- tomato and Mozzarella salad (pages 230–31)
- cucumber and bean-sprout salad (page 231)
- tomato salsa salad (page 232)
- cucumber and mint salad (pages 232–33)

But remember, only one slice of bread per day. So if you intend to have a sandwich for lunch, don't have toast with breakfast.

Lunches prepared at home

Lunches can be prepared at home either as a packed lunch to go or as a meal to be eaten at home. The only real difference between lunch, supper, dinner and late snacks is the size of the meal relative to the time of day; therefore you should look at the following chapters for at-home lunch recipes. The possible variations are infinite – from salmon with lemon butter (see pages 120–21) to prosciutto and courgette frittala (see pages 209–10).

In this book you will notice a significant preponderance of stir-frying. This is a very healthy method of cooking and I cannot recommend it strongly enough. The ingredients are finely sliced, ensuring rapid cooking in a very short period, thereby retaining both the flavour and the nutritional value of the food. And there is the added advantage of a single pan to clean at the end of the meal. Simply perfect!

Chapter 9

Soups

Avocado soup

For 2

50 grams butter

1 medium onion, peeled and diced

1 garlic clove, peeled and finely chopped

1 tbsp plain flour

250 ml chicken stock

1 large, ripe Hass avocado, halved, stoned, peeled and
    chopped

1 tbsp freshly squeezed lemon juice

pinch of rock salt

freshly ground black pepper

60 ml single cream

Heat the butter in a medium frying pan and sauté the onion
and garlic for 1–2 minutes. Remove from the heat and add the
flour, mixing well. Gradually stir in the chicken stock, to ensure
an even consistency. Cook over a low heat for 3–4 minutes.

Add the avocado, lemon juice and chicken stock mixture
to a blender and purée. Season to taste, add almost all of
the cream and blend until smooth. Either chill for 1–2
hours and serve cool, or return to a clean saucepan and
heat gently through – without boiling. This soup is
definitely ruined by overcooking. Pour into bowls and add a
swirl of cream before serving.

Carbohydrate content per serve: 4 grams

Tomato and basil soup

For 2

2 tbsp extra-virgin olive oil

350 grams plum tomatoes, peeled and chopped

1 garlic clove, peeled and finely chopped

3 spring onions, finely chopped

2 tbsp chopped fresh basil

1 bay leaf

350 ml chicken (or vegetable) stock

1 tbsp tomato purée

freshly ground black pepper

2 tsp cornflour

100 ml single cream

pinch of rock salt

2 tsp chopped fresh basil to garnish

A simple method of peeling tomatoes is as follows. Cut a shallow cross through the skin of each tomato at its base. Place the tomatoes in a bowl of boiling water for 30 seconds, then drain off the boiling water. Immerse the tomatoes in cold water for a few seconds, then the skin should peel easily. Ripe tomatoes are *much* easier to peel.

Heat the olive oil in a large saucepan, then add the tomatoes, garlic and spring onions, and cook for 2–3 minutes, stirring frequently. Add the basil, bay leaf, stock and tomato purée. Season with freshly ground black pepper, but do not add further salt at this stage as the stock may be quite salty. Bring to the boil and simmer for 20–30 minutes, then sieve the mixture into a clean saucepan. Make the cornflour into an even paste with a little cold water and add to the soup, mixing evenly. Stir over a low heat until the soup thickens. Add salt to taste (although none may be necessary). Stir in the cream and serve garnished with chopped basil.

Carbohydrate content per serve: **20 grams**

Hot pepper and coriander soup

Perfect served hot for a cold winter's evening, or chilled as a starter.

For 2

2 tbsp extra-virgin olive oil
1 large red pepper, deseeded and diced
1 large red chilli, deseeded and finely chopped
1 garlic clove, peeled and finely chopped
$1/2$ tsp ground turmeric
$1/2$ tsp ground cumin
3 curry leaves
400 ml tomato juice
2 tsp tomato purée
1 tbsp chopped fresh coriander
1 tbsp freshly squeezed lemon juice
pinch of rock salt
freshly ground black pepper
chopped fresh chives, to garnish

Heat the olive oil and sauté the pepper, chilli and garlic for about a minute. Add the ground turmeric, cumin and curry leaves, and cook for a further minute. Stir in the tomato juice, tomato purée, chopped coriander and lemon juice. Season to taste and simmer for 15–20 minutes. Remove the curry leaves, and serve immediately, garnished with chopped fresh chives.

Carbohydrate content per serve: **12 grams**

Carrot and coriander soup

For 2

2 tbsp extra-virgin olive oil
1 medium onion, peeled and finely diced
1 garlic clove, peeled and finely chopped
200 grams of carrots, finely grated
400 ml chicken stock
1 tbsp chopped fresh coriander
2 tsp freshly squeezed lemon juice
pinch of rock salt (optional)
freshly ground black pepper
100 ml single cream
2 tsp chopped fresh chives, to garnish

Heat the olive oil in a medium saucepan and sauté the onion and garlic for about a minute. Add the carrots, mixing well, and sauté on a very low heat for 6–8 minutes. Stir in the chicken stock and coriander. Add the lemon juice, season to taste and simmer for 25–30 minutes. This soup can be puréed; however, I prefer the chunky variety. Stir in the cream and serve immediately, garnished with chopped chives.

Carbohydrate content per serve: **9 grams**

Cream of chicken soup

For 2

50 grams unsalted butter

1 medium onion, peeled and finely diced

1 garlic clove, peeled and finely chopped

1 medium carrot, finely grated

350 ml chicken stock

150 grams cooked skinless chicken breast, finely
  chopped

pinch of rock salt

freshly ground black pepper

1 tbsp chopped fresh chives

1 tbsp chopped fresh basil

150 ml single cream

2 tsp chopped fresh basil leaves, to garnish

Heat the butter in a medium saucepan and sauté the
onion and garlic for about a minute. Stir in the grated
carrot and sauté for a further 2–3 minutes. Add the
chicken stock and chopped chicken, season to taste and
simmer for about 15 minutes. Add the chives and basil,
and blend in a processor until smooth. This can be set
aside until required. Immediately before serving, stir in
the cream and gently heat through, stirring constantly,
but do not allow to boil. Serve immediately, garnished
with chopped fresh basil.

*Carbohydrate content per serve: **5 grams***

Carrot and orange soup

For 2

50 grams unsalted butter

1 medium onion, peeled and finely diced

200 grams of carrots, finely grated

500 ml chicken stock

1 tbsp fresh chopped basil

$^1/_2$ tsp ground nutmeg

juice of a freshly squeezed orange

pinch of rock salt

freshly ground black pepper

2 tbsp single cream

Heat the butter in a medium saucepan and sauté the onion for 2–3 minutes. Stir in the carrots and cook for 4–5 minutes on very low heat. Add the chicken stock, chopped basil, nutmeg and orange juice, and season with to taste. Simmer gently for 20–30 minutes and serve, adding a swirl of fresh cream.

Carbohydrate content per serve: 15 grams

Smoked haddock soup

For 2

2 small smoked haddock fillets

200 ml full-cream milk

1 tbsp chopped fresh chives

1 tbsp chopped fresh dill

1 bay leaf

pinch of rock salt

freshly ground black pepper

50 ml double cream

2 tsp freshly squeezed lemon juice

sprigs of fresh dill to garnish

Roll up the smoked haddock fillets and place them in the base of a saucepan. Pour the milk over the haddock, add the chopped chives, dill, and bay leaf, season with freshly ground black pepper (but not salt at this stage as the smoked haddock can be naturally salty) and simmer over a very gentle heat for about 15 minutes. Remove the bay leaf, add the double cream and lemon juice, and purée in a blender. Return to the heat, check the seasoning, then serve immediately, garnished with dill and a swirl of cream.

Carbohydrate content per serve: **6 grams**

Gazpacho

For 2

1 medium red pepper, deseeded and chopped

1 medium green pepper, deseeded and chopped

1 large green chilli, deseeded and finely chopped

1 garlic clove, peeled and finely chopped

1 Lebanese cucumber, chopped

1 medium red onion, peeled and chopped

400 grams ripe plum tomatoes, peeled and chopped

2 tbsp red wine vinegar

3 tbsp extra-virgin olive oil

300 ml unsweetened tomato juice

2 tsp chopped fresh basil
pinch of rock salt
freshly ground black pepper

Before commencing, set aside a little of the chopped red
and green peppers, cucumber, onion and chilli – sufficient
for garnish later.

Blend the peppers, cucumber, onion, chilli, garlic,
tomatoes, red wine vinegar, olive oil and tomato juice in a
food processor. Season to taste and chill for at least 2 hours
in the fridge. Serve chilled, garnished with the chopped
peppers, cucumber, onion and red chilli.

*Carbohydrate content per serve: **27 grams***

Chapter 10

Fish

Fish can be successfully served at virtually any time of day – from breakfast to supper – and is an essential part of any healthy diet, irrespective of whether you need to lose weight or not. We have already dealt (very briefly) with some possible fish recipes for breakfast. At lunch, we can be a little more adventurous, though obviously time is a constraint on all meals before dinner. Perhaps the easiest – and lightest – dishes are salmon and trout; they are certainly among the richest and most delicious fish on their own merits, and are quite inexpensive in real terms, especially when you consider that you require relatively small portions per person of these rich dishes, and the nutritional value is excellent.

Salmon

Salmon is the perfect meal, with just a simple sauce or salad to enhance its rich flavour. Because it is a fish full of natural oils, it loses none of its flavour by grilling.

Grilled salmon

For 1

1 salmon steak (approximately 2–2.5 cm thick)
1 tbsp extra-virgin olive oil

Brush both sides of the steak with a little olive oil and grill under a hot grill for 3–4 minutes per side, turning once.

Serve immediately with either lightly-steamed mangetout or a simple fresh salad, for example:

- **Rocket and avocado salad**
  See page 233
  Carbohydrate content per serve: 2 grams

- **Cucumber and chive salad**
  See page 234
  Carbohydrate content per serve: 1 gram

- **Tomato, ginger and orange salad**
  See page 234
  Carbohydrate content per serve: 11 grams

Poached salmon

> *Whilst it is quite acceptable to grill rich oily fish, such as salmon, I prefer to retain its delicate flavour and texture by poaching or baking, which I cannot help but believe also retains the nutritional value better than the rather harsher environment of the grill tray. In any event, salmon is equally simple to cook by either method. Allow one salmon steak of about 150 grams per person.*

In a saucepan boil sufficient water to just cover the salmon steaks, then reduce the heat to a gentle simmer. Add a pinch of salt to the water, then lay the fillets in the base of the pan *gently*, and cook for 4–5 minutes. Remove with a fish slice to prevent flaking of the fish, drain and serve on a warm plate with a simple sauce, such as lemon butter sauce (see below).

In the Southern hemisphere, the salmon tends to have a light texture, but a rather bland flavour, and therefore requires sauces for flavour enhancement. However, in the Northern hemisphere, seafood of all varieties has strong and distinctive flavours, and sauces must be light to complement the intrinsic piquancy of the seafood. Salmon has such a rich natural flavour that it requires only the addition of freshly squeezed lemon or lime juice, or a simple lemon and herb butter sauce to complement and accentuate its unique taste to perfection. Several herbs seem to have been developed in nature essentially to accompany fresh salmon!

- **Lemon butter sauce**
For 2
60 grams unsalted butter
juice from ½ a freshly squeezed lemon

Heat the butter in a small saucepan and stir in the freshly squeezed lemon juice. Simmer for 20–30 seconds and serve over the salmon steaks.

Carbohydrate content per serve: 2 grams

- **Lemon and dill butter sauce**
For 2
60 grams unsalted butter
juice from ½ a freshly squeezed lemon
2 tbsp chopped fresh dill

Prepare as above, but add 2 tbsp of chopped fresh dill with the juice of the lemon to the butter, simmer for 30 seconds and serve over the salmon steaks.

Carbohydrate content per serve: **2 grams**

- **Lemon and basil butter sauce**
For 2
60 grams unsalted butter
juice from $\frac{1}{2}$ a freshly squeezed lemon
2 tbsp chopped fresh basil

Prepare as above, substituting 2 tbsp of chopped fresh basil leaves for the dill.

Carbohydrate content per serve: **2 grams**

> *Lightly-steamed (to retain the nutritional value) mangetout or sugar snap peas with yellow squash will complement the flavour and colour of the salmon admirably – with virtually no additional carbohydrate.*

Poached salmon with ginger

> *The words 'salmon' and 'stir-fry' seem to be mutually exclusive – probably because it would be difficult to stir-fry salmon without destroying its delicate texture – but the combination of poached salmon with lightly stir-fried spicy vegetables is both gastronomically delightful, and nutritionally superb!*

For 2

2 salmon steaks, approximately 150–175 grams each

2 tbsp extra-virgin olive oil

3 spring onions, chopped into 3–4 cm lengths

3 slices of fresh ginger root, peeled and finely chopped

1 small red pepper, deseeded and finely sliced

1 small yellow pepper, deseeded and finely sliced

2 tbsp dry sherry

1 tbsp light soy sauce

25 grams raw cashew nuts

25 grams pine nuts

2 tsp freshly squeezed lime juice

pinch of rock salt

freshly ground black pepper

Poach the salmon steaks, as described on page 120.

Heat the olive oil in a wok then sauté the spring onions, ginger and peppers, stirring constantly for 2 minutes. Add the sherry, soy sauce, cashew nuts and lime juice, season to taste and cook for a further 1–2 minutes, then serve with the poached salmon.

*Carbohydrate content per serve: **12 grams***

Salmon with parsley (or dill) sauce

For 2

2 salmon steaks, approximately 150–175 grams each

2 tbsp extra-virgin olive oil

freshly ground black pepper

1 pak choi, washed and halved lengthways

2 sprigs of fresh coriander

Sauce

15 grams plain flour

15 grams butter

150 ml full-cream milk

1 tbsp fresh flat-leaf parsley, finely chopped

Place each salmon steak on a square of aluminium foil, brush lightly with olive oil, add freshly ground black pepper to taste, then close the aluminium parcel and cook in the centre of a pre-heated oven at 180 degrees C (gas mark 4) for 20–25 minutes.

Fill a saucepan with water to a depth of 2–3cm, bring to the boil, then reduce to a gentle simmer and add the pak choi. Cook for 3–4 minutes, turning once.

Heat the butter in a small saucepan. When melted, remove from the heat and gradually stir in the flour. Return to the heat, add the milk gradually, stirring constantly over low heat, until the sauce thickens to an even consistency. Stir in the parsley and add freshly ground black pepper to taste.

Gently open the salmon parcels, remove the salmon steaks with a fish slice and serve on warm plates. Pour the parsley sauce over the salmon steaks, place the pak choi strategically adjacent to the salmon and garnish with sprigs of fresh coriander.

In this recipe, fresh dill can be substituted for fresh parsley.

Carbohydrate content per serve: **10 grams**

Smoked salmon and sour cream salsa

For 2

4 leaves of radicchio lettuce, washed

1 small smoked salmon fillet, sliced finely on the diagonal

pinch of paprika and some fresh basil leaves, to garnish

Sour cream salsa

100 ml sour cream

$^1/_2$ Lebanese cucumber, peeled. Cut 2 slices from the cucumber, then chop the remainder into small cubes

1 tbsp chopped fresh basil

freshly ground black pepper

Mix together the sour cream, chopped cucumber and chopped basil, season with freshly ground black pepper, and set aside to chill in the fridge for 1–2 hours.

Arrange 2 leaves of radicchio lettuce on each plate. Place a slice of cucumber in the centre of the lettuce, and arrange several strips of smoked salmon on the cucumber slice. Spoon a tablespoon of sour cream salsa on the smoked salmon, then add a second layer of smoked salmon and top with another tablespoon of sour cream salsa. Sprinkle with a pinch of paprika and some fresh basil leaves to garnish, and serve immediately or chill in the fridge until required.

Carbohydrate content per serve: 3 grams

Salmon paté

*I have suggested quantities sufficient for four
people in this recipe, as it tastes equally
delicious the next day for breakfast or
lunch.*

For 4

25 grams butter

1 medium onion, peeled and finely diced

1 garlic clove, peeled and finely chopped

200-gram tin of red salmon, bones removed, drained and
   flaked

1 tbsp freshly squeezed lemon juice

1 tbsp dry sherry

1 tbsp chopped fresh flat-leaf parsley

1 large free-range egg, beaten

2 tbsp fine toasted breadcrumbs

50 grams butter, melted

pinch of rock salt

freshly ground black pepper

lemon wedges

sprigs of fresh flat-leaf parsley, to garnish

Heat 25 grams of butter in a small saucepan and sauté the
onion and garlic until softened. Transfer the onion and
garlic to a large mixing bowl, add the salmon, then stir in
the lemon juice, sherry, chopped parsley, egg,
breadcrumbs and melted butter. Season to taste and mix
thoroughly. Line a loaf tin with aluminium foil and press
the salmon paté mixture firmly in the base of the tin.
Close the foil parcel loosely and cook in the centre of a
pre-heated oven at 180 degrees C (gas mark 4) for 45
minutes. Remove and set aside to cool. Serve with a

crispy green salad (pages 229–30) and lemon wedges, garnished with sprigs of fresh flat-leaf parsley.

Carbohydrate content per serve: 16 grams

Trout

Trout is slightly less rich than salmon, but equally delicious in a different way. Because of its intrinsic flavour, it is, like salmon, simple to cook, the basic aim being to avoid spoiling the natural goodness of the food. Trout can similarly be grilled, poached or baked, but again I prefer baking or poaching to retain the nutrition and texture of the fish.

Trout may be substituted for salmon in all of the recipes above. It may be served simply with a squeeze of fresh lemon or lime juice, or with lemon butter (see page 121), lemon and dill butter (see pages 121–22) or lemon and basil butter sauce (see page 122). For some inexplicable reason, the flavour of trout is particularly complemented by nuts – which are an excellent source of vitamin E. It's almost as though nature had planned the gastronomic combination to ensure our continued good health! Trout is usually combined with almonds, which have the dietary advantage of a low carbohydrate content; however, an excellent alternative is pine nuts. The nutritional content is similar and the unique flavours of trout and pine nuts complement one another perfectly. Unlike gastronomic 'experts', I am constrained by the nutritional value and 'dietary potential' of foods. However, in high-quality foods, the dietary potential and nutritional value are virtually identical and effectively equate to the 'taste potential'. Magnificent proteins like fish, meat, poultry and eggs should be enhanced by appropriate natural foods and not overpowered by artificial additives and sauces that detract from the delicious flavours of the foods themselves.

Trout with lemon (or lime) and pine nuts

Trout and pine nuts are a combination made in heaven, both gastronomically and nutritionally. Lemon is not absolutely essential, but it adds a zest that complements the fish, exquisite as this is in splendid isolation! Trout may be grilled in a similar manner to salmon; however, I can see no advantages in this method, either gastronomically or nutritionally. Trout (like most fish) retains nutrients maximally by gentle baking, poaching in a small amount of water, or sautéing in butter with either subtle herb flavours or more simply with lemon or lime juice. What could be simpler, more nutritious or more healthy?

For 2

40 grams butter

2 trout fillets

1 garlic clove, peeled and finely chopped

50 grams pine nuts

juice of a freshly squeezed lemon (or lime)

Heat the butter in a shallow frying pan and gently sauté the trout fillets. Add the garlic, pine nuts and the juice of a freshly squeezed lemon (or lime, depending on personal preference). Cook for approximately 3–4 minutes per side (depending on the size of the fish) and serve with a cucumber and mint salad (pages 232–33).

Carbohydrate content per serve: **9 grams *(including the salad)***

Trout teriyaki

Teriyaki is delicious Japanese sauce, simply and quickly prepared, which perfectly complements the natural flavours of fish, meat or poultry.

For 2

2 trout fillets

3 tbsp sake (Japanese rice wine)

4 tbsp mirin (Japanese sweet wine)

5 tbsp Japanese soy sauce (shoyu), such as tamari – a dark soy sauce. Do not use Chinese soy sauce – it is too strong for this recipe

$^1/_2$ garlic clove, peeled and finely grated

Grate the garlic clove with a small ginger- or garlic-grater.

Mix the sake, mirin, shoyu and garlic, place the trout fillets in a shallow baking dish and pour the marinade over the trout. Cover and chill in the fridge for 6–8 hours, basting with the marinade 2–3 times.

Grill the marinated trout under a pre-heated grill (on high) for 3–4 minutes per side, turning once, and serve immediately.

Carbohydrate content per serve: **6 grams**

Baked trout with ginger and lime

For 2

2 medium trout, cleaned

2 tbsp extra-virgin olive oil

pinch of rock salt

freshly ground black pepper

100 grams sugar snap peas

100 grams French beans

Sauce

2 slices fresh ginger root, peeled and finely chopped

1 tbsp freshly squeezed lime juice

1 garlic clove, peeled and finely chopped

2 tbsp dry sherry

Mix together the ingredients for the sauce in a small bowl.

Wash the trout and pat it dry. Cut three slashes in each side. Place the trout in the centre of individual sheets of aluminium foil, pour the sauce over it, season to taste, then brush it with olive oil. Close the foil *loosely* around the trout. Place the foil parcels on a baking tray in the centre of a pre-heated oven at 180 degrees C (gas mark 4) for 20–25 minutes.

Serve with lightly-steamed sugar snap peas and French beans.

*Carbohydrate content per serve: **8 grams***

Trout with lemon hollandaise sauce

For 2

200 grams washed fresh spinach

2 large rainbow trout, cleaned

40 grams butter, cubed

freshly ground black pepper

wedges of lemon

sprigs of fresh dill, to garnish

Hollandaise sauce

100 grams butter

1 tbsp white wine vinegar

1 tbsp water

$^1/_2$ bay leaf

4 black peppercorns

2 large free-range egg yolks, separated

1 tbsp freshly squeezed lemon juice

pinch of salt

freshly ground black pepper

To prepare the sauce, melt the butter in a medium saucepan and allow to cool. Mix together the white wine vinegar, water, bay leaf and peppercorns in a saucepan, then simmer until the mixture is reduced by half (about 1 tbsp). Sieve, and allow the reduced liquid to cool. Whisk the egg yolks in a heat-safe bowl and beat in the reduced vinegar over simmering water, whisking constantly. When the mixture begins to thicken, slowly add the melted butter, whisking constantly. Add the lemon juice, stirring constantly, season to taste and allow to cool.

Lightly steam the spinach and set aside to cool.

Place the cleaned trout in the base of a shallow oven-proof dish. Dot with the cubes of butter, cover with pierced aluminium foil and cook in the centre of a pre-heated oven at 180 degrees C (gas mark 4) for 20–25 minutes. When cooked, remove the trout from the dish with a perforated fish-slice and set aside to cool. Then carefully peel off the skin and place the trout on a bed of steamed spinach. Season with freshly ground black pepper, pour the lemon hollandaise sauce over the trout and serve with a lemon wedge, garnished with sprigs of fresh dill.

Carbohydrate content per serve: 1 gram

Lemon sole with pak choi

For 2

4 lemon sole fillets
2 pak choi, halved lengthways
2 tbsp light soy sauce
1 tsp sesame oil
2 tsp fresh coriander, finely chopped
pinch of rock salt
freshly ground black pepper
sprigs of fresh coriander, to garnish

Place the lemon sole fillets in a lightly-buttered, shallow oven-safe dish, sprinkle with 1 tsp chopped fresh coriander, add sufficient water to just cover the base of the dish, cover and cook in a pre-heated oven at 180 degrees C (gas mark 4) for 12–15 minutes, depending on the size of the fillets.

Whilst the lemon sole fillets are cooking, add water to a large saucepan, to a depth of about 3 cm, bring to the boil, then reduce the heat to a gentle simmer. Lay the pak choi halves in the boiling water, cover and simmer for 2–3 minutes, turning once. Remove the pak choi with a perforated spoon.

Mix together the soy sauce, sesame oil and 1 tsp chopped fresh coriander.

Remove the cooked lemon sole fillets from the baking dish with a fish slice and place on warm plates. Arrange the pak choi halves on the plate and drizzle over the sauce. Garnish with sprigs of fresh coriander.

Carbohydrate content per serve: **negligible**

Dover sole with herb sauce

For 2

2 Dover sole

15 grams butter

15 grams plain flour

150 ml full-cream milk

1 tbsp chopped fresh dill

1 tsp chopped fresh chervil

1 tsp chopped fresh flat-leaf parsley

1 tsp freshly squeezed lemon juice

pinch of rock salt

freshly ground black pepper

fresh chervil, to garnish

Brush the Dover sole with melted butter and cook under a hot grill for about 8–10 minutes, turning once.

Melt the butter in a small saucepan. Remove from the heat, add the flour and beat to a smooth consistency. Return to a low heat and gradually mix in the milk, constantly stirring to maintain an even consistency. Stir in the chopped dill, chervil, parsley and lemon juice, season to taste and cook for about 2 minutes, stirring constantly.

Serve the sauce over the sole and garnish with fresh chervil.

*Carbohydrate content per serve: **11 grams***

Tuna with herbs

For 2

4 tbsp extra-virgin olive oil
300 grams fresh tuna, cubed
1 large red onion, peeled and finely sliced
1 garlic clove, peeled and finely chopped
1 medium red pepper, deseeded and chopped
1 medium green pepper, deseeded and chopped
400-gram tin of plum tomatoes, ready-peeled and chopped
1 tbsp chopped fresh coriander
1 tbsp chopped fresh basil
1 bay leaf
1 tbsp tomato purée
75 ml dry white wine
pinch of rock salt
freshly ground black pepper
chopped fresh chives, to garnish

Heat 3 tablespoons of the olive oil in a large frying pan and brown the tuna on medium heat. Remove the tuna with a perforated spoon, set aside and cover.

Add the remaining tablespoon of olive oil to the pan, stir in the onion, garlic and peppers, and sauté for 1–2 minutes, then add the plum tomatoes (with the juice), herbs, bay leaf, tomato purée and white wine. Simmer for 4–5 minutes, stirring frequently. Return the tuna to the pan, season to taste and simmer for 4–5 minutes. Remove the bay leaf and serve, garnished with chopped fresh chives.

Carbohydrate content per serve: **14 grams**

Tuna in dill mayonnaise with mangetout

For 2

200-gram tin of tuna in brine (or springwater), drained
1 tbsp chopped fresh dill
freshly ground black pepper
100 grams French beans
100 grams mangetout
50 grams rocket
Parmesan shavings and fresh dill, to garnish

Mayonnaise

2 free-range egg yolks, separated
1 tbsp freshly squeezed lemon juice
1 tsp Dijon mustard
1 tsp white wine vinegar
250 ml extra-virgin olive oil

To prepare mayonnaise, all ingredients *must* be at room temperature. Blend the egg yolks, lemon juice, mustard and white wine vinegar to a smooth consistency using a whisk or blender. Gradually – and *very slowly* – add the olive oil whilst stirring, and blend until smooth.

Steam the French beans and mangetout.

Mix 1 tablespoon of the mayonnaise, the tuna and the chopped fresh dill in a bowl and season with freshly ground black pepper. Serve with the French beans and mangetout on a base of rocket and garnish with freshly ground black pepper, shavings of Parmesan cheese and fresh dill.

Carbohydrate content per serve: **6 grams**

Tuna burrito

In this recipe, commercial mayonnaise can be substituted for home-made (although it doesn't taste as good), but check that it does not have hidden carbohydrates. A good mayonnaise contains a negligible amount of carbohydrate and is therefore ideal for this diet. This recipe allows one tortilla per person; as tortillas contain between 20 and 25 grams of carbohydrate each (depending on the manufacturer), no other bread should be consumed that day.

For 2

200-gram tin of tuna (in brine or springwater), drained and flaked

1 tbsp mayonnaise

1 tbsp chopped fresh basil

1 tbsp chopped fresh chives

pinch of rock salt

freshly ground black pepper
2 medium flour tortillas
small handful of curly endive lettuce
2 vine-ripened tomatoes, chopped

Mix together the tuna, mayonnaise, basil, chives and seasoning in a medium bowl.

Wrap the tortillas in aluminium foil and warm in a hot oven for 1 minute.

Spoon a quarter of the tuna mayonnaise mixture on to each tortilla. Place some curly endive lettuce and chopped tomato on the tuna, add a further layer of tuna mayonnaise, top with a final layer of endive lettuce and tomato, and season with freshly ground black pepper. Close the tortilla and serve.

Carbohydrate content per serve: 22–27 grams (including 20–25 grams for the tortilla)

Cod with basil and chives

For 2

2 cod steak fillets (approximately 150–175 grams each)
1 tbsp chopped fresh chives
25 grams butter, cubed
pinch of rock salt
freshly ground black pepper
3 tbsp extra-virgin olive oil
1 medium onion, peeled and chopped
1 garlic clove, peeled and finely chopped
125 grams button mushrooms, wiped

1 small red pepper, deseeded and sliced
1 small orange pepper, deseeded and sliced
2 medium courgettes, sliced lengthways into quarters
1 tbsp fresh basil, finely chopped
2 tbsp dry sherry
chopped almonds, to garnish

Place the cod steaks in the base of a casserole dish, sprinkle over the chives and dot with butter. Season to taste, cover with pierced aluminium foil and bake in the centre of a pre-heated oven at 180 degrees C (gas mark 4) for 12–15 minutes.

Heat the olive oil in a wok and sauté the onion and garlic for about a minute, then add the mushrooms, peppers, courgettes, basil and sherry. Cook for 2-3 minutes, stirring frequently.

Serve the sauce over the cod steaks and garnish with chopped almonds.

Carbohydrate content per serve: **11 grams**

Cod with tomato and coriander salsa

For 2

2 cod steaks, approximately 150 grams each
1 tbsp extra-virgin olive oil
tomato and coriander salsa (see page 232)
pinch of rock salt
freshly ground black pepper
fresh coriander leaves, to garnish

Brush the cod steaks with the olive oil and grill on a high heat for 6–7 minutes, turning once. Season to taste and serve on warm plates with the tomato and coriander salsa, garnished with fresh coriander.

Carbohydrate content per serve: **7 grams**

Cod with parsley sauce

A classic recipe – which is also perfect for a low-carbohydrate diet.

For 2

2 cod steaks, approximately 150 grams each
15 grams unsalted butter
15 grams plain flour
150 ml full-cream milk
1 tbsp chopped fresh flat-leaf parsley
freshly ground black pepper
fresh flat-leaf parsley, to garnish
150 grams baby leeks

Place the cod steaks in the base of a buttered, shallow, oven-safe dish, add sufficient water to just cover the base of the dish, cover and bake in the centre of a pre-heated oven at 180 degrees C (gas mark 4) for 12–14 minutes. Remove from the oven and place the cod steaks on warm plates.

While the cod is baking, heat the butter in a small saucepan, then remove from the heat and gradually stir in the flour. Return to a low heat and gradually add the milk, stirring constantly. When the mixture reaches an even consistency and is just beginning to thicken, remove from the heat and mix in the parsley. Season with freshly ground black pepper and pour over the cod steaks.

Lightly steam the baby leeks and serve with the cod. Garnish with fresh flat-leaf parsley.

*Carbohydrate content per serve: **12 grams***

Swordfish steaks with lemon and garlic

For 2

2 swordfish steaks, approximately 150 grams each
juice of a freshly squeezed lemon
1 garlic clove, peeled and grated
25 grams unsalted butter, cubed
lemon wedges
sprigs of fresh dill, to garnish

Place the swordfish steaks in the base of a shallow oven-safe casserole dish, squeeze the juice of half a fresh lemon over each steak, sprinkle over the grated garlic and dot with cubes of butter. Cover with pierced aluminium foil, place in the centre of a pre-heated oven at 180 degrees C (gas mark 4) and cook for 15–20 minutes. Serve with a tomato and avocado salad (pages 222–23), garnished with lemon wedges and sprigs of fresh dill.

*Carbohydrate content per serve: **12 grams** (including the salad)*

Mackerel

Mackerel is a very rich fish, high in essential omega-3 fatty acids and vitamin D. It is an acquired taste, and people seem to either love it or loathe it. If you haven't tried mackerel, please do. For some reason, which I have never understood, it is not one of the most popular fish, but it is certainly one of the most tasty and nutritious.

Smoked mackerel paté

For 2

1 smoked mackerel fillet
2 tbsp sour cream
50 grams Philadelphia cream cheese
1 tbsp chopped fresh chives
1 tsp freshly squeezed lemon juice
pinch of rock salt
freshly ground black pepper
pinch of cayenne pepper and some lemon zest, to
    garnish

Flake the smoked mackerel to remove all bones and skin. Put it in a blender with the sour cream, cream cheese, chopped chives and lemon juice. Season to taste, and purée until smooth. Transfer to a medium bowl and chill for 2–3 hours before serving.

Serve the smoked mackerel paté with a crispy green salad (see pages 229–30), garnished with a pinch of cayenne pepper and some lemon zest.

*Carbohydrate content per serve: **5 grams (including salad)***

Grilled mackerel with lime

For 2

2 mackerel fillets

juice of a freshly squeezed lime

freshly ground black pepper

2 tbsp extra-virgin olive oil

lime wedges

Squeeze the juice of half a lime over each fillet and season with freshly ground black pepper. Although mackerel is very rich in natural oils, I prefer to brush it with olive oil to retain all of the nutrients. Place under a medium grill for 3–4 minutes per side, turning once, and serve with lime wedges, either alone or with cucumber and beansprout salad (see page 231).

Carbohydrate content per serve: **5 grams**

Mackerel with lemon and coriander

For 2

2 mackerel fillets

juice of a freshly squeezed lemon

1 tbsp chopped, fresh coriander

25 grams unsalted butter, cubed

lemon wedges

$^1/_2$ tbsp fresh coriander leaves, to garnish

Place the mackerel fillets in the base of a shallow, oven-safe casserole dish, squeeze over them the juice of half a lemon and sprinkle on the chopped fresh coriander. Arrange the butter cubes evenly over the mackerel, then cover with pierced aluminium foil and cook in the centre of a pre-heated oven at 180 degrees C (gas mark 4) for 15–18 minutes. Serve with lemon wedges, garnish with fresh coriander leaves and serve with rocket and olive salad (see pages 225–26)

Carbohydrate content per serve: **3 grams**

Smoked mackerel with crushed black pepper

Smoked mackerel is such a rich dish, full of natural flavours, that it requires very little accompaniment. Crushed black peppercorns complement the richness of the mackerel perfectly.

For 2

2 smoked mackerel fillets
8–10 black peppercorns, crushed
2 tbsp extra-virgin olive oil
100 grams French beans
sprigs of fresh dill, to garnish

Brush the mackerel fillets on both sides with extra-virgin olive oil and coat the fillets with the crushed peppercorns. Place under a hot grill and cook for 3–4 minutes per side, turning once.

Serve with lightly steamed French beans and garnish with sprigs of fresh dill.

Carbohydrate content per serve: **3 grams**

Whiting with ginger and lime

For 2

2 tbsp extra-virgin olive oil

2 shallots, peeled and finely diced

1 garlic clove, peeled and finely chopped

4 whiting fillets, approximately 75–80 grams each

75 grams butter

2 tsp freshly squeezed lime juice

$1/2$ tsp freshly grated lime rind

2 slices fresh ginger, peeled and grated

1 tbsp chopped fresh dill

pinch of rock salt

freshly ground black pepper

lime wedges

sprigs of fresh dill, to garnish

150 grams sugar snap peas

100 grams button mushrooms, wiped and halved

Heat the olive oil in a large frying pan and sauté the diced shallots and garlic.

Lightly sauté the whiting fillets, turning once.

Melt the butter in a small saucepan; stir in the lime juice, lime rind, and fresh ginger, and gently heat for 1–2 minutes. Add the chopped dill and season to taste. Transfer the whiting fillets to warm plates, spoon the sauce over the fillets and garnish with sprigs of fresh dill and lime wedges.

Steam the sugar snap peas and sauté the mushrooms in butter. Serve with the whiting.

*Carbohydrate content per serve: **7 grams***

Soused herrings with radish and basil salad

*It is difficult to think of a more nutritious –
and underutilized – fish than herring. Packed
with protein, omega-3 essential fatty acids
and vitamin D, it's a fast food with body!*

For 2

4 herring fillets
pinch of rock salt
freshly ground black pepper
225 ml white wine vinegar
75 ml water
6–8 peppercorns
1 bay leaf
1 tsp granulated sugar
1 clove

Season the herring fillets with salt and freshly ground black pepper and roll them from head to tail, with the skin outside. Mix the white wine vinegar and water. Place the herrings in an oven-safe dish, pour over just enough of the vinegar mixture to cover the herring, and add the peppercorns, bay leaf, sugar and clove. Cook in the centre of a pre-heated oven at 180 degrees C (gas mark 4) for 15 minutes.

Serve on a bed of sweet Romaine lettuce with radish and basil salad (see page 228).

Carbohydrate content per serve: 8 grams (including salad)

Haddock with peppers and ginger

For 2

2 tbsp extra-virgin olive oil

1 red onion, peeled and diced

1 garlic clove, peeled and finely chopped

2 slices of fresh root ginger, peeled and finely chopped

1 small red pepper, deseeded and finely sliced

1 small green pepper, deseeded and finely sliced

1 small yellow pepper, deseeded and finely sliced

1 tbsp chopped fresh dill

1 tbsp chopped fresh chervil

pinch of rock salt

freshly ground black pepper

2 large haddock fillets, approximately 150 grams each

25 grams butter, melted

1 tbsp chopped fresh chives, to garnish

Heat the olive oil in a wok and sauté the onion and garlic for about a minute. Add the ginger, peppers, chervil and dill, and season to taste. Stir-fry for 2–3 minutes, stirring frequently.

Spoon the vegetables on to two large aluminium foil rectangles, lay the haddock fillets on the bed of vegetables, brush with melted butter and season with freshly ground black pepper. Close the aluminium parcels loosely, then cook in the centre of a pre-heated oven at 180 degrees C (gas mark 4) for about 15 minutes. Serve in the opened parcels, garnished with freshly chopped chives.

Carbohydrate content per serve: 10 grams

Poached haddock with mushroom and sherry sauce

For 2

2 large haddock fillets, approximately 125–150 grams
    each

pinch of rock salt

freshly ground black pepper

2 tsp freshly squeezed lemon juice

200 ml full-cream milk

2 tbsp extra-virgin olive oil

75 grams button mushrooms, wiped and sliced

1 tbsp sweet sherry

15 grams butter

15 grams plain flour

150 ml full-cream milk

1 tbsp chopped fresh chives

fresh coriander leaves, to garnish

Place the haddock fillets in a single layer in the base of a
shallow oven-safe dish, season with salt and freshly ground
black pepper, and drizzle over 2 tsp of freshly squeezed
lemon juice. Add sufficient milk to just cover the haddock.
Cover with pierced aluminium foil and place in the centre
of a pre-heated oven at 180 degrees C (gas mark 4) for
about 15 minutes. Remove the haddock with a perforated
fish slice, and place on warm plates.

In the meantime, heat the olive oil in a medium
saucepan and sauté the mushrooms for 1–2 minutes, then
stir in the sherry. Remove the mushrooms from the heat
and set aside.

Melt the butter in a separate small saucepan, remove
from the heat and stir in the flour, mixing to a smooth

consistency. Return to the heat and gradually stir in 150 ml of milk. Return to a low heat, stirring constantly until the sauce thickens. Remove from the heat and gradually add the mushrooms to the sauce, stirring constantly. Stir in the chopped chives and heat gently before pouring over the poached haddock. Garnish with fresh coriander leaves.

Carbohydrate content per serve: **18 grams**

Chapter 11

Shellfish

Shellfish are an individual taste: people seem either to love or loathe shellfish, but there can be no denying their superb nutritional value.

Incidentally, you will notice that 'tiger prawns' can include a variety of different species of different sizes, from Crevettes (at 6-8 cm) to larger specimens up to 15 cm, depending on the fishmonger. In the following recipes, tiger prawns are the 6–8 cm variety.

Prawns in garlic butter

Easy and quick to prepare, this recipe tastes delicious and is nutritionally superb, with virtually no carbohydrate content. Simply perfect!

For 2

300 grams raw tiger prawns, shelled
3 tbsp extra-virgin olive oil
2 garlic cloves, peeled and finely chopped
chopped fresh coriander, to garnish

The easiest way to shell a prawn is to break off the head and tail, remove the legs, and the shell will then peel off easily and quickly. Using a sharp knife – and great care – slice down the back of the prawn and devein the dark thread by washing under running water.

Heat the extra-virgin olive oil and sauté the garlic for

approximately 30–40 seconds. Add the peeled prawns and cook – stirring regularly – for 3–4 minutes, depending upon the size of the prawns, until cooked. Remove the prawns from the pan and cover.

Prepare a garlic butter sauce according to the recipe on page 163, pour over the prawns and garnish with fresh, chopped coriander.

Carbohydrate content per serve: **negligible**

Tiger prawn salad with avocado lime dressing

For 2

300 grams cooked tiger prawns, shelled and deveined

1 tbsp freshly squeezed lime juice

3 tbsp dry white wine

100 grams mixed curly green lettuce leaves (curly endive, mizuna, cos and green coral)

2 spring onions, chopped into 4–5 cm lengths

lime zest, to garnish

Dressing

1 small ripe Hass avocado, halved, stoned and diced

2 shallots, peeled and chopped

1 tbsp freshly squeezed lime juice

2 tbsp extra-virgin olive oil

freshly ground black pepper

Marinate the cooked tiger prawns, lime juice and white wine for 2–3 hours in the fridge.

Blend the avocado, shallots, lime juice, olive oil and

freshly ground black pepper (either with a blender or by hand) until smooth.

Mix the lettuce leaves and spring onions in a large salad bowl, arrange the tiger prawns on the lettuce and spoon the avocado dressing on the salad. Garnish with lime zest.

Carbohydrate content per serve: **4 grams**

Tiger prawns with basil and tomatoes

For 2

2 tsp sesame seeds

2 tbsp extra-virgin olive oil

3 spring onions, peeled and chopped into 4–5 cm lengths

1 garlic clove, peeled and finely chopped

1 small red pepper, deseeded and finely sliced

200 gram tin of plum tomatoes, chopped

2 tsp tomato purée

1 tbsp sweet sherry

pinch of rock salt

freshly ground black pepper

250 grams cooked tiger prawns, shelled and deveined

1 tbsp fresh basil, finely chopped

sprigs of fresh oregano, to garnish

Lightly toast the sesame seeds and set aside.

Heat the olive oil in the wok until hot, add the spring onions and garlic, and sauté for 1–2 minutes. Add the sliced red pepper and cook for a further minute, stirring frequently, then add the tomatoes, tomato purée and sherry, and season to taste. Simmer for 1–2 minutes. Finally, add the pre-cooked tiger prawns and chopped basil, and simmer gently for a further 4–5 minutes. Serve immediately, garnished with fresh oregano and sesame seeds.

*Carbohydrate content per serve: **9 grams***

Prawns and avocado

For 2

1 ripe Hass avocado, halved, stoned, peeled and finely diced
4 large vine-ripened tomatoes, peeled and finely chopped
2 spring onions, finely chopped
150 grams frozen cooked prawns, thawed
pinch of rock salt
freshly ground black pepper
75 ml mayonnaise
1 tbsp chopped fresh chives

Dressing

1 tbsp white wine vinegar
4 tbsp extra-virgin olive oil
1 tbsp freshly squeezed lemon juice
1 tsp Dijon mustard

Mix together the white wine vinegar, olive oil, lemon juice and mustard in a screw-top jar.

Mix the avocado, tomatoes, spring onions and prawns in

a large bowl, drizzle over the dressing, season to taste and toss gently. Top with freshly made mayonnaise (see page 135), and garnish with chopped chives.

*Carbohydrate content per serve: **10 grams***

Hot and spicy prawns

For 2

2 tbsp extra-virgin olive oil

3 spring onions, chopped into 4–5cm lengths

1 garlic clove, peeled and finely chopped

2 tsp plain flour

100 ml fish stock

2 tsp Worcestershire sauce

2 tsp lemon juice

2 tsp tomato purée

4–5 drops of Tabasco sauce

1 bay leaf

pinch of rock salt

freshly ground black pepper

1 small orange pepper, deseeded and sliced

1 small yellow pepper, deseeded and sliced

1 tbsp chopped fresh coriander

250 grams cooked and peeled tiger prawns

fresh coriander leaves, to garnish

Heat the extra-virgin olive oil in a wok and sauté the spring onions and garlic. Remove from the heat and stir in the flour. Gradually stir in the fish stock, then add the Worcestershire sauce, lemon juice, tomato purée, Tabasco sauce and bay leaf. Season to taste and simmer for 2–3 minutes, stirring frequently. Add the peppers, coriander and pre-cooked tiger prawns, and simmer for a further 4–5 minutes. Remove the bay leaf before serving, and garnish with fresh coriander leaves.

Carbohydrate content per serve: 11 grams

Prawns with rocket salad

For 2

3 tbsp extra-virgin olive oil

250 grams cooked prawns

handful of rocket leaves

1 small ripe Hass avocado, halved, stoned, peeled and finely sliced

freshly ground black pepper

1 tbsp chopped chives

lime wedges

Sauce

100 grams unsalted butter

2 tsp freshly squeezed lemon juice

freshly ground black pepper

1 tbsp chopped fresh chives

1 tbsp chopped fresh chervil

1 tbsp chopped fresh basil

Melt the butter in a small saucepan and stir in the lemon juice, freshly ground black pepper, chives, chervil and basil.

Heat the olive oil in a saucepan and sauté the prawns for 2–3 minutes. Remove from the pan and cover.

Arrange the avocado slices like the spokes of a wheel, centred in the middle of the plate. Place the rocket leaves on the avocado and season with freshly ground black pepper. Place the cooked prawns on the rocket and pour the herb butter sauce over them. Serve with lime wedges and garnish with chopped chives.

Carbohydrate content per serve: **2 grams**

Chilli tiger prawns with mangetout

For 2

2 tbsp extra-virgin olive oil
1 garlic clove, peeled and finely chopped
2 spring onions, chopped into 4–5 cm lengths
100 grams mangetout
1 small green chilli, deseeded and finely chopped
250 grams cooked tiger prawns, peeled and deveined
1 tbsp sweet sherry
pinch of rock salt
freshly ground black pepper
sesame oil
chopped fresh chives, to garnish

Heat the olive oil and sauté the garlic, spring onions, mangetout, and chilli for about 2 minutes. Add the cooked tiger prawns and sherry. Season to taste and stir-fry for another 2 minutes, stirring frequently. Serve on warm plates, drizzle over a few drops of sesame oil and garnish with freshly chopped chives.

Carbohydrate content per serve: **6 grams**

Scallops with lime and ginger

For 2

250 grams fresh scallops, cleaned

3 tbsp extra-virgin olive oil

100 grams mangetout

3 shallots, peeled and quartered

1 garlic clove, peeled and grated

2 slices of fresh ginger root, peeled and finely chopped

1 small red pepper, deseeded and finely sliced

75 grams button mushrooms, wiped and halved

freshly ground black pepper

lime wedges

fresh tarragon, to garnish

Marinade

2 tbsp light soy sauce

1 tbsp sweet sherry

1 slice fresh ginger root, peeled and finely chopped

1 garlic clove, peeled and grated

1 tbsp freshly squeezed lime juice

1 tsp cornflour

Mix together the ingredients of the marinade, add the scallops and marinate in the fridge for 2–3 hours.

Heat 2 tablespoons of the olive oil in a wok, add the scallops and sauté gently for about 3 minutes. Remove the scallops with a perforated spoon, set aside and cover. Heat the remaining olive oil in the wok, add the mangetout, shallots, garlic, ginger and red pepper, and cook for 2 minutes, stirring frequently. Return the scallops to the wok, add the mushrooms, and season with freshly ground black pepper. Cook on medium heat for another 3 minutes and serve with wedges of lime, garnished with fresh tarragon.

Carbohydrate content per serve: **12 grams**

Scallops and asparagus with sweet chilli sauce

Scallops and asparagus complement one another wonderfully in every respect: taste, texture and nutritional content. This recipe has extra zest – and vitamins – when fresh chilli is included; however, it is still delicious and nutritious without chilli, for those who prefer life less hot!

For 2

1 bunch of fresh asparagus, trimmed and chopped into
    5–6 cm lengths

3 tbsp extra-virgin olive oil

1 garlic clove, peeled and finely chopped

2 shallots, finely chopped

250 grams cleaned, fresh scallops

1 small red chilli, deseeded and finely chopped
    (optional)

2 tbsp light soy sauce

2 tbsp sweet sherry

$1/2$ tsp granulated sugar

30 grams melted butter

freshly ground black pepper

fresh coriander leaves, to garnish

Lightly steam the asparagus, transfer to a warm plate and cover.

Heat the extra-virgin olive oil in the wok and sauté the garlic, shallots, scallops and chilli over medium heat for 3–4 minutes. Add the soy sauce, sherry, sugar and melted butter, season with freshly ground black pepper, and cook for a further 2 minutes. Arrange the asparagus aesthetically on warm plates, serve the chilli scallops on the asparagus and garnish with fresh coriander leaves.

*Carbohydrate content per serve: **4 grams***

Ginger scallops with mangetout

For 2

3 tbsp extra-virgin olive oil

250 grams fresh, cleaned scallops

1 garlic clove, peeled and finely chopped

3 slices of fresh ginger root, peeled and finely chopped

100 grams of mangetout

1 small red pepper, deseeded and finely sliced

1 tbsp light soy sauce

2 tbsp freshly squeezed orange juice

freshly ground black pepper

chopped fresh chives, to garnish

Heat the extra-virgin olive oil in the wok, add the scallops and sauté for 2–3 minutes. Remove the scallops carefully (to prevent breaking) with a perforated spoon. Add the garlic and ginger to the wok, and stir-fry for 30–40 seconds, then add the mangetout and pepper, and sauté for a further 2 minutes. Return the scallops to the wok, add the soy sauce and orange juice, stir gently and cook for a final 2–3 minutes. Serve garnished with chopped fresh chives.

*Carbohydrate content per serve: **7 grams***

Mussels in tomato sauce with oregano

For 2

750 grams fresh mussels, bearded and scrubbed
2 tbsp extra-virgin olive oil
4 baby onions, peeled
1 garlic clove, peeled and finely chopped
2 tbsp tomato purée
100 ml dry white wine
400-gram tin of chopped plum tomatoes
1 tbsp chopped fresh oregano
fresh oregano, to garnish

Wash and scrub the mussels, discarding any open or damaged mussels.

Heat the olive oil in a large saucepan and sauté the baby onions and garlic for 1–2 minutes. Add the tomato purée, white wine and tomatoes (plus juice). Stir in the mussels and oregano, bring to the boil, then cover and simmer on high heat for 5–7 minutes. Discard any unopened mussels and serve immediately, garnished with fresh oregano.

*Carbohydrate content per serve: **14 grams***

Mussels in garlic sauce

For 2

750 grams fresh mussels, bearded and scrubbed

2 tbsp fresh thyme, finely chopped

1 medium onion, peeled and diced

pinch of rock salt

freshly ground black pepper

150 ml dry white wine

100 grams butter

4 garlic cloves, peeled and grated

sprigs of fresh thyme, to garnish

Wash and scrub the mussels several times, discarding any that are open. When you are completely satisfied regarding the safety of the mussels, place them in a large saucepan with the chopped thyme, onion, salt, freshly ground black pepper and wine. Bring to the boil, then cover and simmer on a high heat until the mussels open (usually 5–7 minutes); remember only to use those which have opened. Remove the opened mussels with a perforated spoon and transfer to a shallow casserole dish. Cover and place in the centre of a warm oven. Strain the mixture, return the remaining liquid to the pan and reduce by about half. Add the butter and finely grated garlic, simmer gently for 2–3 minutes and pour over the mussels. Garnish with sprigs of fresh thyme.

Carbohydrate content per serve: 4 grams

Chapter 12

Meat

Red meat can be a problem at the moment, with BSE and the recent foot and mouth epidemic – and we are now told that pork may also have been contaminated with BSE. But then, salmonella has been reported in poultry and eggs, chemicals are used by some fishermen to bleach fish fillets 'white', and some vegetables are genetically-modified. Unfortunately you have no alternative but to take some risk with your food. I'm certainly not saying that interfering with nature is correct; on the contrary, I consider it immoral, but virtually every food currently available seems to have some man-made risk so we may as well continue to consume a balanced diet, as best we can.

It is very important in a diet of this nature to include foods cooked in the most natural manner, because these foods have natural flavours and nutrition which simply cannot be reproduced by artificial procedures. And whilst we can – and will – add nutritious sauces and accompaniments, it is essential to bear in mind that the meat (or fish, or poultry, or shellfish) is the real star of the meal; the sauces will (hopefully) enhance, but merely play the supporting role in the meal.

Grilled pepper steak with French beans

For 2

2 sirloin or fillet steaks, about 150 grams each, and no
    more than 2.5 cm thick
2 tbsp extra-virgin olive oil
freshly ground black pepper
100 grams French beans

Brush the steaks with olive oil on both sides and season
liberally with freshly ground black pepper. Place under a
hot grill, at least 8 cm from the source of heat, and grill to
taste, turning once.

Steam the French beans until tender but still firm. The
French beans can be simply served with the steaks or with
one of the sauces below.

Carbohydrate content per serve: **negligible**

- **Lemon butter sauce**
  60 grams unsalted butter
  juice of ¹/₂ a freshly squeezed lemon
  freshly ground black pepper

Heat the butter in a small saucepan, stir in the lemon juice
and freshly ground pepper, to taste, and serve .

Carbohydrate content per serve: **2 grams**

- **Garlic butter sauce**

  75 grams unsalted butter

  2 garlic cloves, peeled and grated

  1 tsp chopped flat-leaf parsley

  1 tsp lemon juice

  freshly ground black pepper

Heat the butter in a small saucepan, stir in the garlic, parsley, lemon juice and freshly ground black pepper, and serve.

Carbohydrate content per serve: 2 grams

- **Ginger and oyster sauce**

  1 tbsp extra-virgin olive oil

  2–3 drops sesame oil

  1 garlic clove, peeled and finely chopped

  1 tsp oyster sauce

  2 slices of fresh ginger root, peeled and finely chopped

  1 tbsp sweet sherry

  2 tbsp water

  freshly ground black pepper

Heat the olive oil and sesame oil in a small saucepan, add the garlic and sauté for about a minute. Add the oyster sauce, ginger root, sherry and water and cook on medium heat for approximately 2 minutes, stirring frequently. Serve.

Carbohydrate content per serve: 4 grams

Sirloin steak with Stilton cheese

For 2

2 sirloin steaks, about 150 grams each
2 tbsp extra-virgin olive oil
50 grams Stilton cheese, crumbled
pinch of rock salt
freshly ground black pepper
1 tsp chopped fresh chives, to garnish

Brush the steaks with olive oil, then grill under medium heat according to individual taste (3–4 minutes per side is usually adequate). Season to taste, top with crumbled Stilton cheese, then place under the grill until the cheese melts. Serve immediately, garnished with freshly chopped chives.

Carbohydrate content per serve: **negligible**

Beef casserole with chives

Tinned tomatoes are deliberately utilised in this dish, as they seem to provide an even richer source of lycopene (that marvellous antioxidant) than do fresh tomatoes.

Beef casserole can be served with numerous accompaniments, but fresh green vegetables are undoubtedly most nutritious and complementary. Try lightly steamed broccoli florets, fresh peas, French beans, spinach or mangetout; the average serving only adds about 2–4 grams of carbohydrate to the meal.

Although casseroles and stews are made

*with cheaper cuts of meat, the nutritional
value is the same as that of more expensive
cuts. But you do have to cook the meat longer,
and therefore it involves a little more forward-
planning. The dishes taste equally delicious,
in a different way with the blending of
individual flavours during cooking.*

For 2

400 grams blade or round steak, chopped into large cubes
pinch of rock salt
2 tsp dry English mustard
freshly ground black pepper
1 tbsp plain flour
50 grams butter
2 large onions, peeled and chopped
1 large garlic clove, peeled and finely chopped
1 large carrot, peeled and sliced
400-gram tin of plum tomatoes, ready-peeled
200 ml beef stock
2 tbsp chopped fresh chives

Coat the steak with flour, then mix it with the salt, dry
mustard and freshly ground pepper in a large bowl.

Heat the butter and sauté the onions and garlic for
approximately 1–2 minutes, or until soft. Add the meat and
brown for 2–3 minutes. Then gradually blend in the carrot,
tomatoes (including the juice) and stock, and season to
taste. Spoon into a casserole dish, cover and cook for about
2 hours at 180 degrees C or gas mark 4. Serve topped with
freshly-chopped chives.

*Carbohydrate content per serve: **21 grams***

Moussaka

For 2

1 large fresh aubergine, sliced

pinch of rock salt

3 tbsp extra-virgin olive oil

1 large onion, peeled and finely chopped

1 medium garlic clove, peeled and finely chopped

250 grams beef mince

3 large plum tomatoes, peeled and chopped

1 tbsp tomato purée

75 ml beef stock

freshly ground black pepper

Sauce

15 grams butter

15 grams plain flour

150 ml full-cream milk

50 grams grated cheese (preferably, but not essentially,
Greek Kefalotyri)

freshly ground black pepper

Clean and slice the aubergine, then arrange in salted layers in a colander for 30 minutes. Rinse thoroughly and pat dry. Arrange the aubergine slices in a single layer on a baking tray, brush with a thin layer of olive oil and cook in a pre-heated oven at 180 degrees C (gas mark 4) for 10 minutes. Remove from the oven and set aside to cool.

Heat 2 tablespoons of the olive oil and sauté the onion and garlic for 1–2 minutes until soft, then add the minced beef, stirring regularly until evenly browned. Add the chopped tomatoes and tomato purée, and stir in the stock. Season to taste and gently simmer for 10–15 minutes.

Arrange half the aubergine slices in the base of an oven-proof casserole dish, add the beef mixture, then top with a second layer of aubergine slices.

To prepare the sauce, heat the butter in a saucepan until melted, remove from the heat and gradually mix in the flour, stirring constantly. Return to a low heat and slowly add the milk, stirring constantly. When the mixture has reached an even consistency, add the grated cheese and stir until evenly melted into the sauce. Season to taste.

Pour the sauce over the mixture in the casserole dish, top with a little grated cheese and bake in a pre-heated oven for 35–40 minutes at 180 degrees C (gas mark 4).

Serve with Feta salad (see pages 223–24).

Carbohydrate content per serve: **27 grams (including salad)**

Beef stroganoff

For 2

4 tbsp extra-virgin olive oil
1 large onion, peeled and finely sliced
1 garlic clove, peeled and finely chopped
75 grams button mushrooms, wiped and halved
1 tbsp plain flour
pinch of rock salt
freshly ground black pepper
250 grams fillet steak, sliced in thin strips
1 tsp tomato purée
100 ml beef stock
1 tbsp chopped fresh basil
1 tbsp chopped fresh parsley

100 ml sour cream

1 tbsp chopped fresh chives, to garnish

Heat 2 tablespoons of the extra-virgin olive oil in a large pan and sauté the onion and garlic for approximately 1 minute. Add the mushrooms and sauté for a further minute. Transfer to a casserole dish, cover and place in a warm oven, 140 degrees C (gas mark 1).

Coat the steak in seasoned flour.

Heat the remaining olive oil in the pan and brown the steak, stirring regularly. Return the onion, garlic and mushrooms to the pan, and add the stock, tomato purée and fresh herbs. Simmer for 12–15 minutes, remove from the heat and stir in the sour cream. Serve immediately, garnished with chopped fresh chives.

Carbohydrate content per serve: 12 grams

Sliced beef in oyster sauce

For 2

250 grams steak, sliced into thin strips

3 tbsp extra-virgin olive oil

1 garlic clove, peeled and finely chopped

2 slices of fresh ginger root, peeled and finely chopped

100 grams mushrooms, wiped and halved (the dish will have a better aesthetic appearance if you use a mixture of different mushrooms, but the nutritional value is the same for all mushrooms)

4 spring onions, chopped into 3–4-cm lengths

100 grams broccoli florets

1 small red pepper, deseeded and finely sliced
$1/2$ tsp granulated sugar
freshly ground black pepper
1 green chilli, deseeded and cut into strips, to garnish
   (optional)

Marinade
1 tbsp light soy sauce
1 tbsp oyster sauce
1 tbsp sweet sherry
1 tsp cornflour

Mix the soy sauce, oyster sauce, sherry and cornflour to an even consistency, then add to the sliced beef in a large bowl. Marinate in the fridge for 3–4 hours.

Heat 2 tablespoons of the extra-virgin olive oil in the wok and stir-fry the beef for 2 minutes. Add the ginger and garlic and cook for a further 2 minutes, stirring constantly. Remove from the wok with a perforated spoon and set aside.

Heat the remaining olive oil in the wok, add the mushrooms, broccoli, spring onions and red pepper, and stir-fry for 2–3 minutes. Return the beef to the wok, add the oyster sauce marinade and sugar, and stir-fry for a further 2–3 minutes. Season with freshly ground black pepper and serve garnished with green chilli strips.

Carbohydrate content per serve: **16 grams**

Steak and asparagus

For 2

2 sirloin or fillet steaks, about 150 grams each, and no
  more than 2.5 cm thick
1 tbsp extra-virgin olive oil
freshly ground black pepper
200 grams fresh asparagus

Brush the steaks with olive oil, season with freshly ground
black pepper and grill to taste, turning once.

Lightly steam the asparagus until tender but firm. Serve
with one of the following sauces.

Carbohydrate content per serve: **negligible**

- **Lemon butter sauce**
  (See page 162)
Carbohydrate content per serve: **2 grams**

- **Herb butter sauce**
  75 grams unsalted butter
  1 tsp chopped fresh chives
  1 tsp chopped fresh rosemary
  pinch of paprika
  1 tsp freshly squeezed lemon juice
  freshly ground black pepper

Melt the butter in a small saucepan, then stir in the chives,
rosemary, paprika and lemon juice. Season with freshly
ground black pepper and serve over the asparagus.

Carbohydrate content per serve: **2 grams**

Pot-roast beef

*Simple to prepare, and full of flavour and
nutrition. This recipe provides an excellent
meal for four people, or dinner for two and
sufficient roast beef for lunch the following day.*

For 4

1 kilogram rolled brisket of beef
4 tbsp extra-virgin olive oil
2 medium onions, peeled and chopped
1 garlic clove, peeled and finely chopped
1 tbsp plain flour
500 ml beef stock
200 grams carrots, peeled and sliced on the diagonal
100 grams swede, peeled and cubed
1 bay leaf
1 tbsp fresh flat-leaf parsley, finely chopped
2 tsp tomato purée
1 tsp dry mustard
pinch of rock salt
freshly ground black pepper
sprigs of fresh flat-leaf parsley, to garnish

Heat the olive oil in a large saucepan and brown the brisket
of beef *thoroughly* on all sides. Remove the beef from the
pan (leaving the juices in the pan), place in a large
casserole dish and cover.

Add the onions and garlic to the pan and sauté for 1–2
minutes. Stir in the flour, then gradually stir in the stock.
Add the remainder of the vegetables and simmer for a
further 3–4 minutes. Stir in the bay leaf, parsley, tomato
purée, and mustard. Season to taste, then add to the
casserole dish, mixing well. Cover and place in the centre

of a pre-heated oven at 140 degrees C (gas mark 1) for about 2 hours. Ovens vary, so you should test the meat to ensure that it is tender, and return it to the oven for a further 30 minutes if necessary. Remove the bay leaf before serving and garnish with fresh flat-leaf parsley.

*Carbohydrate content per serve: **17 grams***

Goulash

For 2

2 tbsp plain flour

1 tbsp paprika

pinch of rock salt

freshly ground black pepper

250 grams of casserole steak, chopped into 4–5-cm cubes

2 tbsp extra-virgin olive oil

1 large onion, peeled and chopped

1 garlic clove, peeled and finely chopped

200-gram tin of plum tomatoes, chopped

2 tsp tomato purée

150 ml beef stock

2 tsp chopped fresh dill

2 tsp chopped fresh thyme

2 tsp chopped fresh parsley

100 ml sour cream

sprigs of fresh thyme, to garnish

Mix the flour with the paprika and season with salt and freshly ground black pepper. Coat the steak in the seasoned flour. Heat 2 tbsp of olive oil in a frying pan and brown the steak. Add the onion and garlic and sauté for about 1 minute. Add the tomatoes, tomato purée, stock and herbs, stirring constantly. Season to taste and simmer for about an hour. Stir in the sour cream and serve immediately, garnished with sprigs of fresh thyme.

*Carbohydrate content per serve: **21 grams***

Beef chop suey

You can substitute similar quantities of lean pork, chicken breast, or peeled and pre-cooked prawns for beef in this dish, and a vegetarian version is equally successful.

For 2

250 grams lean steak, thinly sliced

3 tbsp extra-virgin olive oil

1 garlic clove, peeled and finely chopped

3 spring onions, chopped into 4–5-cm lengths

1 carrot, sliced lengthways into matchsticks

1 yellow pepper, deseeded and thinly sliced

75 grams mangetout

75 grams bean sprouts

2 slices fresh ginger root, peeled and finely chopped

2 tbsp light soy sauce

1 tsp granulated sugar

pinch of rock salt

freshly ground black pepper

Heat 2 tablespoons of the extra-virgin olive oil in a wok, then stir-fry the steak for 2–3 minutes, stirring frequently. Remove from the wok with a perforated spoon, set aside and cover.

Heat the remaining tablespoon of olive oil in the wok, add the garlic, spring onions, carrot, pepper and mangetout, and stir-fry for 1–2 minutes. Then add the bean sprouts, ginger, soy sauce, sugar and seasoning, and cook for another 1–2 minutes, stirring frequently. Return the steak to the wok and stir-fry for 2 minutes, then serve on warm plates.

Carbohydrate content per serve: 12 grams

Beef kebabs

For 2

250 grams lean steak, cubed

1 large red pepper, deseeded and chopped into 3-cm cubes

12 button mushrooms, wiped and trimmed

1 large green pepper, deseeded and chopped into 3-cm cubes

12 yellow squash

freshly ground black pepper

3 tbsp extra-virgin olive oil

2 tbsp chopped fresh chives, to garnish

Marinade

2 tbsp dry sherry

1 tbsp light soy sauce

1 garlic clove, peeled and finely chopped

1 slice of fresh ginger root, peeled and finely chopped

1 tsp freshly squeezed lemon juice

1 tsp honey

pinch of rock salt
freshly ground black pepper

Marinate the steak for 2–3 hours. Soak the wooden skewers in water for a similar period.

Thread the steak, peppers, button mushrooms and squash on the skewers. Brush with extra-virgin olive oil and season with freshly ground black pepper, then grill (or barbecue) until the meat is cooked to taste. Garnish with chopped fresh chives, and serve with a cucumber and bean-sprout salad (see page 231).

Carbohydrate content per serve: 11 grams (including salad)

Cabernet Sauvignon beef

For 2

300 grams casserole steak, chopped into 4–5-cm cubes
2 tbsp plain flour
pinch of rock salt
freshly ground black pepper
3 tbsp extra-virgin olive oil
300 ml Cabernet Sauvignon red wine
1 garlic clove, peeled and finely chopped
1 bay leaf
1 tsp tomato purée
1 tbsp chopped fresh thyme
1 tbsp chopped fresh sage
25 grams butter
8 baby onions, peeled
100 grams button mushrooms, wiped and halved

75 grams carrots, julienned
75 grams French beans
75 grams broccoli florets

Coat the steak in seasoned flour, heat the olive oil in a large frying pan and brown the steak. Slowly add the Cabernet Sauvignon, and stir in the garlic, bay leaf, tomato purée, thyme and sage. Season to taste and transfer to an oven-safe casserole dish.

In a separate pan, melt the butter and sauté the onions and mushrooms lightly. Transfer the onions and mushrooms to the casserole dish and stir gently. Cover, and cook in the centre of a pre-heated oven for 2 hours at 140 degrees C (gas mark 1).

Serve with lightly steamed carrots, French beans and broccoli florets.

Carbohydrate content per serve: 22 grams

Sweet and sour pork

For 2
2 tbsp plain flour
pinch of rock salt
freshly ground black pepper
250 grams lean pork fillet, sliced thinly on the diagonal
3 tbsp extra-virgin olive oil
4 spring onions, chopped into 4–5-cm lengths
1 garlic clove, peeled and finely chopped
1 small red pepper, deseeded and finely sliced
1 small yellow pepper, deseeded and finely sliced
1 tsp granulated sugar

10 ml white wine vinegar

50 ml pork stock

1 tsp tomato purée

1 tbsp light soy sauce

1 tbsp sweet sherry

finely chopped spring onion, to garnish

Coat the pork with seasoned flour.

Heat 2 tablespoons of the olive oil in the wok and stir-fry the pork over a medium heat for 4–5 minutes, stirring frequently. Remove the pork with a perforated spoon, set aside and cover.

Heat the remaining tablespoon of olive oil in the wok. Reduce the heat to medium and sauté the spring onions and garlic for about a minute, then add the red and yellow peppers, and stir-fry for 2–3 minutes. Return the pork to the wok, stir in the sugar, white wine vinegar, stock, tomato purée, soy sauce, and sherry. Simmer for about 3–4 minutes and serve immediately, garnished with finely chopped spring onion.

*Carbohydrate content per serve: **21 grams***

Pork with ginger

For 2

250 grams lean pork fillet, sliced thinly on the diagonal

3 tbsp extra-virgin olive oil

1 garlic clove, peeled and finely chopped

3 slices of fresh ginger root, peeled and finely chopped

100 grams mangetout

3 spring onions, chopped into 4–5-cm lengths

1 medium carrot, peeled and chopped into matchsticks
pinch of rock salt
freshly ground black pepper

Marinade
2 tbsp light soy sauce
1 tsp cornflour
2 tbsp dry sherry

Mix the soy sauce and sherry in a large bowl and stir in the
cornflour to ensure an even consistency. Add the pork and
marinate in the fridge for at least 2 hours.

Heat 2 tablespoons of the olive oil in a wok and stir-fry
the pork for 2–3 minutes, stirring frequently. Remove the
pork with a perforated spoon, set aside and cover.

Heat the remaining tablespoon of olive oil in the wok,
add the garlic, ginger, mangetout, spring onions and carrot.
Season to taste, stir-fry for 2–3 minutes, then return the
pork to the wok. Cook for another 2 minutes and serve
immediately.

Carbohydrate content per serve: **10 grams**

Pork chops with herbs

For 2
3 tbsp dry white wine
1 garlic clove, peeled and finely chopped
1 tsp chopped fresh sage
1 tsp chopped fresh rosemary
2 large pork chops
2 tbsp extra-virgin olive oil

4 green olives, finely sliced

1 tsp chopped flat-leaf parsley

Mix together the white wine, garlic, sage and rosemary, add the pork chops and marinate in the fridge for 3–4 hours.

Heat the olive oil in a large frying pan and cook the pork chops for 2–3 minutes per side on medium heat. Pour the remainder of the marinade over the pork, and cook for another 2–3 minutes, turning once. Garnish with olives and chopped fresh parsley, and serve with cucumber and bean-sprout salad (see page 231).

Carbohydrate content per serve: 1 gram

Spicy lamb

For 2

350 grams lean lamb fillet, cubed

3 tbsp extra-virgin olive oil

2 green cardamom pods

1 cinnamon stick

1 clove

2 bay leaves

1 medium onion, peeled and finely sliced

1 garlic clove, peeled and finely chopped

2 slices of fresh ginger root, peeled and finely
   chopped

1 tbsp chopped fresh coriander

$1/2$ tsp chilli powder

$1/2$ tsp ground cumin

200-gram tin plum tomatoes, chopped into large
   segments

1 tbsp tomato purée
150 ml lamb stock

Marinade
150 ml natural yoghurt
pinch of rock salt
freshly ground black pepper
1 garlic clove, peeled and finely chopped
1 tbsp freshly squeezed lemon juice

Mix together the yoghurt, salt, pepper, garlic and lemon juice. Stir in the lamb and marinate in the fridge for at least 4–6 hours, preferably overnight.

Heat the olive oil in a large frying pan and sauté the cardamom pods, cinnamon stick and clove for about 2 minutes. Add the bay leaf and onion, and sauté until softened. Add the garlic, ginger, coriander, chilli powder and ground cumin, mix well, and cook for approximately 2 minutes. Add the lamb to the pan and stir-fry for 4–5 minutes, then add the chopped tomatoes, tomato purée and stock. Bring to the boil, then reduce heat to a gentle simmer. Cover and simmer gently for approximately 1 hour. Remove the bay leaves, cinnamon stick and cardamom pods, and serve with a crispy green salad (see pages 229–30).

Carbohydrate content per serve: **19 grams**

Lamb skewers with cucumber raita

*Once again, a delicious and nutritious meal
with virtually no carbohydrate (so there is no
restriction on quantity). Who said dieting was
difficult?*

For 2

300 grams lean minced lamb

1 medium onion, peeled and grated

1 tbsp chopped fresh coriander

1 garlic clove, peeled and grated

1 tbsp chopped fresh flat-leaf parsley

half tsp ground cumin

$1/2$ small green chilli, deseeded and finely chopped

1 egg white, separated

pinch of rock salt

freshly ground black pepper

lime wedges

fresh coriander leaves, to garnish

Cucumber raita

150 ml natural yoghurt

1 tbsp chopped fresh mint leaves

1 small Lebanese cucumber, finely chopped

Grate the garlic with a ginger- or garlic-grater.

Mix together the lamb, onion, coriander, garlic, parsley,
cumin, chilli, egg white and seasoning (to taste) in a large
bowl. Mould the lamb mixture into a sausage shape around
kebab sticks, pressing firmly, then cool in the fridge for 2–3
hours. This will help to retain the kebabs' shape whilst
grilling.

Mix the chopped fresh mint and cucumber with the

yoghurt, and cool in the fridge for 2–3 hours.

Remove the kebabs from the fridge and grill on a high heat for 5–7 minutes, turning once. Serve with the mint yoghurt dressing and lime wedges, and garnish with fresh mint leaves.

Carbohydrate content content per serve: 8 grams

Lamb curry with red pepper

For 2

4 tbsp extra-virgin olive oil
2 medium onions, peeled and chopped
1 garlic clove, peeled and finely chopped
2 small red peppers, deseeded and finely sliced
1 bay leaf
2 green cadamom pods
350 grams lean lamb fillet, cubed
1 tsp garam masala
1 slice fresh ginger root, peeled and finely chopped
1 green chilli, seeded and finely chopped
1 tbsp freshly squeezed lemon juice
200-gram tin of chopped plum tomatoes (not drained)
200 ml lamb stock
4 tbsp natural yoghurt
1 tbsp fresh coriander, finely chopped
pinch of rock salt
freshly ground black pepper
fresh coriander leaves and slices of red chilli, to garnish

Heat the extra-virgin olive oil in a large, deep frying pan and sauté the onions, garlic, red peppers, bay leaf and

cardamom pods for 1–2 minutes. Add the lamb and sauté
for a further 4–5 minutes. Stir in the garam masala, ginger,
chilli, lemon juice and tomatoes, and cook for 2–3 minutes.
Stir in the stock and simmer gently for 45 minutes. Remove
the bay leaf and cardamom pods, then stir in the yoghurt
gradually over low heat. Finally, add the fresh coriander,
season to taste and simmer over low heat for a further 3–4
minutes. Serve immediately, garnished with fresh
coriander leaves and finely sliced red chilli.

Carbohydrate content per serve: 16 grams

Lamb kebabs with sour cream and chive sauce

For 2

300 grams lean lamb fillet, cubed

6 small pickling onions, peeled

6 cherry tomatoes

12 small button mushrooms, wiped

1 yellow pepper, deseeded and chopped into large
  pieces

1 green pepper, deseeded and chopped into large
  pieces

6 skewers

2 tbsp extra-virgin olive oil

freshly ground black pepper

lime wedges

Sauce

100 ml sour cream

50 grams Lebanese cucumber, finely diced

2 tsp chopped fresh chives
1 garlic clove, peeled and finely grated
1 tsp lemon juice

Place the sour cream, cucumber, chives, garlic and lemon juice in a medium bowl and mix thoroughly. Chill in the fridge for 2 hours before serving.

Chop the peppers into segments about the size of the lamb cubes, to ensure even cooking times. Thread the lamb cubes, onions, tomatoes, button mushrooms and segments of peppers aesthetically on to 8 skewers. (If wooden skewers are used, remember to soak the skewers in cold water for at least 2 hours before use.) Brush the lamb and vegetables with the olive oil, season with freshly ground black pepper and grill under a hot grill (or barbecue) for 10–12 minutes, turning frequently. Serve with the chilled sour cream sauce and lime wedges.

*Carbohydrate content per serve: **12 grams***

Roast lamb

Roast meats provide delicious hot meals, and equally delicious cold meals the next day. The meat cooks itself with very little preparation, and is really another example of a perfect fast food – except that it is also healthy!

For 4

Leg of lamb (about 1¹/₂ kg)
pinch of rock salt
freshly ground black pepper
2 garlic cloves, peeled and sliced

3 tbsp extra-virgin olive oil

2 tbsp chopped fresh rosemary

sprigs of fresh mint to garnish

150 grams French beans

150 grams carrots, peeled and sliced lengthways into
matchsticks (Julienne)

150 grams courgettes, Julienne

Season the lamb with salt and freshly ground black pepper
to taste. Slash the lamb lightly and insert garlic slices into
the cuts. Brush the joint with olive oil, sprinkle freshly
chopped rosemary over it, place it in a buttered roasting
pan and cook in the centre of a pre-heated oven at 220
degrees C (gas mark 7) for 20 minutes. Reduce the
temperature to 190 degrees C (gas mark 5) and continue to
cook according to the following formula: 20 minutes for
each 450 grams, plus an additional 10 minutes. Remove
from the oven, allow to cool before carving and garnish
with fresh mint.

Lightly steam the French beans, carrots and courgettes, and
serve with the lamb.

Carbohydrate content per serve: **9 grams**

Chilli lamb

For 2

250 grams lean lamb fillets, sliced into thin strips

3 tbsp extra-virgin olive oil

1 tsp sesame oil

1 small red chilli, deseeded and finely chopped

3 spring onions, chopped into 4–5-cm lengths
2 slices of fresh ginger root, peeled and grated
1 garlic clove, peeled and finely chopped
1 small red pepper, deseeded and finely sliced
1 small orange pepper, deseeded and finely sliced
50 grams sugar snap peas
2 tbsp light soy sauce
2 green courgettes, chopped on the diagonal
freshly ground black pepper
pinch of rock salt

Heat 2 tablespoons of the olive oil in a wok and stir-fry the lamb until tender. Remove from the pan with a perforated spoon, pat dry and set aside to cool.

Heat the remaining olive oil and sesame oil in the wok, add the chilli, spring onions, ginger, garlic, peppers, sugar snap peas and soy sauce, and stir-fry for 1–2 minutes. Return the lamb to the wok, add the courgettes, season to taste, stir-fry for a further 2–3 minutes and serve.

Carbohydrate content per serve: **7 grams**

Stir-fried lamb with ginger

For 2

200 grams lean lamb fillet, thinly sliced
3 tbsp extra-virgin olive oil
3 spring onions, chopped into 4–5-cm lengths
1 garlic clove, peeled and finely chopped
3 slices of fresh ginger root, peeled and finely chopped
1 medium carrot, Julienne

1 medium yellow pepper, deseeded and finely sliced
100 grams mangetout
pinch of rock salt
freshly ground black pepper

Marinade
2 tbsp light soy sauce
1 tbsp dry sherry
1 tsp granulated sugar
half a garlic clove, peeled and finely chopped
1 slice of fresh ginger root, peeled and finely chopped
2 tsp cornflour

In a medium bowl mix together the soy sauce, sherry, sugar, garlic and ginger, and gradually stir in the cornflour to an even consistency.

Marinate the lamb for 2–3 hours, stirring occasionally.

Heat 2 tablespoons of the olive oil in the wok, then stir-fry the lamb for 2–3 minutes. Remove with a perforated spoon and cover.

Heat the remaining tablespoon of olive oil, add the spring onions, garlic, ginger, carrot, pepper and mangetout, and stir-fry for 2–3 minutes. Return the lamb to the wok, season to taste and stir-fry for a further 2 minutes.

Carbohydrate content per serve: **16 grams**

Liver with sour cream

Liver is not a popular dish today, which is incredible when one considers how nutritious and tasty it is. Our forebears of only 30 years ago would be astounded if you tried to convince them that liver was off the menu simply because it was no longer trendy! Liver is a marvellous dish; try it and see. It is packed full of protein, vitamins and minerals; for example, there is 3–4 times more vitamin C in liver than in the equivalent weight of citrus fruits.

For 2

4 thin slices of lamb's liver (approximately 250 grams),
   sliced into strips
2 tbsp plain flour
1 tbsp paprika
pinch of rock salt
freshly ground black pepper
3 tbsp extra-virgin olive oil
1 large onion, peeled and chopped
1 garlic clove, peeled and finely chopped
200-gram tin of plum tomatoes, chopped
2 tsp tomato purée
150 ml beef stock
2 tsp chopped fresh thyme
2 tsp chopped fresh coriander
2 tsp chopped fresh basil
100 ml sour cream
sprigs of fresh thyme, to garnish

Mix the flour with the paprika and season with salt and

freshly ground black pepper. Coat the liver in the seasoned flour. Heat the extra-virgin olive oil in a frying pan and brown the liver. Add the onion and garlic and sauté for about 1 minute. Add the tomatoes, tomato purée, stock and herbs, stirring constantly. Season to taste and simmer for about 30 minutes. Stir in the sour cream and serve immediately, garnished with sprigs of fresh basil.

Carbohydrate content per serve: **21 grams**

Braised liver with mushrooms

For 2

2 tbsp plain flour
pinch of rock salt
freshly ground black pepper
4 thin slices of lamb's liver (approximately 250 grams)
4 tbsp extra-virgin olive oil
1 garlic clove, peeled and finely chopped
1 large onion, peeled and chopped
1 tbsp sweet sherry
150 grams of button mushrooms, wiped and halved
1 bay leaf
sprigs of fresh thyme, to garnish

Season the flour with the salt and black pepper and coat the liver with it.

Heat 3 tablespoons of the olive oil in a frying pan, then cook the liver for about 6 minutes, turning once. Remove with a perforated spoon to a shallow dish, cover and place in a warm oven. Heat the remaining tablespoon of olive oil in the pan and sauté the onion and garlic for about a minute. Add the sherry, mushrooms and bay leaf, and sauté for a further 2 minutes. Return the liver to the pan and cook on medium heat for 2 minutes, turning once. Remove the bay leaf and serve, garnished with fresh thyme.

*Carbohydrate content per serve: **16 grams***

Liver casserole

For 2

2 tbsp plain flour
pinch of rock salt
freshly ground black pepper
3–4 slices of lamb's liver (about 250–300 grams)
3 tbsp extra-virgin olive oil
1 medium onion, peeled and finely sliced
1 garlic clove, peeled and finely chopped
1 green pepper, deseeded and chopped into large
  segments
1 large carrot, peeled and sliced on the diagonal
3 tbsp dry white wine
200 ml lamb stock
1 tsp chopped fresh thyme
1 tsp chopped fresh flat-leaf parsley

Season the flour with the salt and black pepper and coat the liver with it.

Heat 2 tablespoons of olive oil in a large pan and brown the liver. Remove the liver with a perforated spoon, place in a casserole dish and cover.

Add the remaining tablespoon of olive oil to the pan and sauté the onion and garlic for approximately 1 minute. Add the green pepper and carrot, and sauté for a further 2 minutes, stirring frequently. Stir in the wine and stock, chopped fresh thyme and parsley, and season to taste. Transfer to the casserole dish, cover and cook in a pre-heated oven at 140 degrees C (gas mark 1), for about 2–2$^{1}/_{2}$ hours, depending on the oven.

Carbohydrate content per serve: **20 grams**

Lamb's liver with herbs

For 2

3 tbsp extra-virgin olive oil

1 medium red onion, peeled and diced

1 garlic clove, peeled and finely chopped

4 thin slices of lamb's liver (approximately 250 grams)

2 tbsp plain flour

pinch of rock salt

freshly ground black pepper

200-gram tin plum tomatoes

1 tbsp chopped fresh oregano

1 tbsp chopped fresh basil

1 tbsp chopped fresh chives

100 grams sugar snap peas

100 grams yellow squash

Heat 2 tablespoons of the extra-virgin olive oil in a large frying pan and sauté the onion and garlic for 1–2 minutes. Coat the liver with seasoned flour, heat the remaining olive oil and cook the liver for 5–6 minutes on medium heat,

turning once. Add the tomatoes, oregano and basil, season
to taste, and simmer for 5–7 minutes. Serve with lightly
steamed sugar snap peas and yellow squash, garnished with
chopped fresh chives.

Carbohydrate content per serve: **22 grams**

Chapter 13

Poultry

Tandoori-style chicken

For 2

2 skinless chicken breasts (about 150 grams each), or 6
    chicken drumsticks, skin removed

100 ml natural yoghurt

1 garlic clove, peeled and grated

1 slice of fresh ginger root, peeled and grated

1 tsp garam masala

1 tsp ground paprika

$^1/_2$ tsp ground turmeric

$^1/_2$ tsp ground coriander

$^1/_4$ tsp ground cumin

2 tbsp freshly squeezed lemon juice

pinch of rock salt

freshly ground black pepper

lemon wedges

Cut two slits in each of the chicken pieces (breast or
drumsticks). Mix the yoghurt with the garlic, ginger, spices,
lemon juice and seasoning, and coat the chicken with the
sauce. Marinate in the fridge for at least 4 hours (preferably
overnight).

Lay the chicken in a single layer on an oven tray, cover
with pierced aluminium foil and cook in the centre of a pre-
heated oven for 30–35 minutes at 180 degrees C (gas mark
4), turning once.

Serve with a crispy green salad (see pages 229–30) and lemon wedges.

*Carbohydrate content per serve: **11 grams***

Ginger chicken with orange

For 2

3 tbsp extra-virgin olive oil

2 skinless chicken breasts (approx 125–150 grams each), sliced into thin strips

3 slices fresh ginger root, peeled and finely chopped

4 shallots, peeled and sliced

1 garlic clove, peeled and finely chopped

1 small red pepper, deseeded and finely sliced

1 sweet orange (preferably Valencia), peeled, centre pith and pips removed, and segmented

chopped fresh chives, to garnish

Sauce

2 tbsp light soy sauce

1 tbsp honey

1 tsp cornflour

100 ml fresh orange juice

Mix the soy sauce, honey and orange juice in a medium bowl, then stir in the cornflower and mix to an even consistency.

Heat 2 tablespoons of the olive oil in a wok and sauté the sliced chicken breast for about 2–3 minutes. Add the ginger and cook for a further 2–3 minutes. Remove from the wok with a perforated spoon and set aside. Heat the remaining tablespoon of olive oil in the wok, then add the shallots, garlic and red pepper. Stir-fry for about 2 minutes, then return the chicken and ginger to the wok. Stir in the honey and orange soy sauce, and cook on a high heat for a further 2 minutes. Add the orange segments, stir gently, then serve immediately (or the orange segments will disintegrate), garnished with chopped chives.

*Carbohydrate content per serve: **26 grams***

Chicken tikka

A delicious dish, not too spicy, which combines the natural proteins, vitamins and minerals of the chicken with the vitamins and antioxidants of the herbs.

For 2

300 grams skinless chicken breast, cubed

Marinade

1/2 tsp chilli powder

1 garlic clove, peeled and finely chopped

2 slices fresh ginger root, peeled and finely chopped

1/2 tsp ground turmeric

1/2 tsp ground cumin

1 shallot, peeled and grated

pinch of rock salt

freshly ground black pepper

2 tsp fresh lemon juice

100 ml natural yoghurt

2 tsp fresh coriander, finely chopped

Mix together the chilli powder, garlic, ginger, turmeric, cumin, shallot, salt, pepper, lemon juice, natural yoghurt and coriander in a medium bowl, and stir in the chicken. Cover and leave to marinate in the fridge for at least 3–4 hours – or preferably overnight.

Grill the marinated chicken under medium heat for about 20 minutes, turning regularly.

Serve with a crispy green salad (see pages 229–30) and lime wedges.

*Carbohydrate content per serve: **11 grams***

Lemon chicken with cashew nuts

For 2

3 tbsp extra-virgin olive oil

250 grams skinless chicken breast, thinly sliced

50 grams raw cashew nuts

lemon wedges

lemon zest to garnish

75 grams mangetout

75 grams broccoli florets

Sauce

1 tsp cornflour

2 tbsp water

juice of a freshly squeezed lemon

1 tbsp light soy sauce

2 tbsp sweet sherry

Prepare the cornflour mixture by adding the cornflour to 2 tablespoons of water, stirring to ensure an even consistency.

Heat the olive oil in the wok, then stir-fry the chicken breast strips on medium heat for about 3–4 minutes, stirring frequently. Remove the chicken to a casserole dish, mix with the cashew nuts, cover and place in a warm oven. Drain the wok and wipe clean.

Mix together the lemon juice, soy sauce and sherry in a bowl, and stir in the cornflour paste, mixing to an even consistency. Transfer to the wok and heat to a gentle simmer, stirring constantly for about 1–2 minutes, until the sauce thickens.

Return the chicken and cashew nuts to the wok and simmer for 2–3 minutes.

Lightly steam the mangetout and broccoli florets. Garnish the chicken with lemon zest and serve with the vegetables.

Carbohydrate content per serve: 15 grams

Chicken with prosciutto

Some cooks believe it is heretical to mix meat with poultry. Fortunately, I am a doctor, not a cook! My excuse is that the correct combination can be nutritionally superb and taste divine. This dish can be quickly prepared for either lunch or supper.

The cheese in this recipe can be varied according to taste – it is equally delicious with Edam, Emmental, Gruyere or Jarlsberg. I consider strong cheeses (such as some cheddars and Stilton) to be too overpowering for this combination. If you are partial to

> cheeses with strong flavour (which I think are
> wonderful in other circumstances), then
> simply reduce the quantity.

For 2

2 skinless chicken breast fillets (about 150 grams each)
2 tbsp plain flour, seasoned
2 tbsp extra-virgin olive oil
1 tbsp chopped fresh basil, finely chopped
4 large slices of prosciutto (sliced)
30 grams freshly grated Parmesan cheese
freshly ground black pepper
1 tsp chopped fresh chives, to garnish
1 tsp chopped fresh coriander, to garnish

Using a sharp knife, slice each chicken breast lengthways
into two thin, flat halves. Season the flour with salt and
black pepper and lightly coat the chicken breasts with it.
Heat the olive oil in a frying pan, add the chicken fillets
and chopped basil, and cook over a moderate heat for 8–10
minutes, turning twice, until evenly cooked on both sides.
Remove the chicken to a grill-pan, place a slice of
prosciutto on each fillet, and sprinkle grated Parmesan
cheese on the prosciutto. Season with freshly ground black
pepper and place under a pre-heated grill until the cheese
has just melted.

Serve with tomato and avocado salad (see pages 222–23),
garnished with fresh chives and coriander.

*Carbohydrate content per serve: **20 grams (including salad)***

Chicken korma

For 2

300 grams skinless chicken breasts, cubed

3 tbsp extra-virgin olive oil

2 green cardamom pods

1 medium onion, peeled and finely chopped

1 garlic clove, peeled and finely chopped

1 slice of fresh ginger root, peeled and finely chopped

1 tsp ground cumin

$1/2$ tsp garam masala

$1/2$ tsp chilli powder

pinch of rock salt

freshly ground black pepper

125 ml natural yoghurt

pinch of paprika and some fresh coriander leaves, to
garnish

Heat 2 tablespoons of the olive oil in a large frying pan and
sauté the chicken for 5–6 minutes, stirring frequently.
Remove the chicken with a perforated spoon, place it in a
casserole dish and cover.

Heat the remaining tablespoon of olive oil in the pan,
add the cardamom pods, onion and garlic, and sauté for 2–3
minutes. Remove from the heat and stir in the ginger,
cumin, garam masala, chilli powder and seasoning. Cook
over a low heat for 2–3 minutes, stirring constantly. Stir in
the yoghurt gradually, simmer over low heat for 2–3
minutes, then return the chicken to the pan. Heat through
gently for about 3–4 minutes, then serve, garnished with a
pinch of paprika and some fresh coriander leaves.

Carbohydrate content per serve: **7 grams**

Spicy chicken drumsticks

For 2

6 chicken drumsticks, skin removed

25 grams unsalted butter, cubed

Marinade

1 garlic clove, peeled and finely grated

1 tbsp Worcestershire sauce

1 tbsp tomato purée

$\frac{1}{2}$ tsp granulated sugar

3–4 drops Tabasco sauce

1 tsp freshly squeezed lemon juice

pinch of rock salt

freshly ground black pepper

Mix together the garlic, Worcestershire sauce, tomato purée, sugar, Tabasco sauce, lemon juice and seasoning, and marinate the chicken drumsticks in the fridge for 2 hours.

Place the drumsticks in a single layer in the base of a shallow, oven-proof dish and pour the remainder of the marinade over the drumsticks. Arrange the butter cubes evenly over the chicken, cover with pierced aluminium foil and place in the centre of a pre-heated oven at 180 degrees C (gas mark 4) for 35–40 minutes. Serve with rocket and olive salad (see pages 225–26).

Carbohydrate content per serve: **6 grams** *(including salad)*

Chicken with tomato and basil sauce

For 2

2 skinless chicken breasts (about 150 grams each)
25 grams butter, cubed
3 tbsp extra-virgin olive oil
1 medium onion, peeled and chopped
1 garlic clove, peeled and finely chopped
400-gram tin of plum tomatoes
1 tbsp tomato purée
50 ml dry white wine
75 ml chicken stock
75 grams of button mushrooms, wiped and halved
1 tbsp chopped fresh basil
pinch of rock salt
freshly ground black pepper
fresh basil leaves to garnish
100 grams broccoli florets
100 grams carrots, julienned

Place the chicken breasts in the base of a shallow casserole tray, arrange the cubes of butter on the chicken, then cover with pierced aluminium foil and cook in centre of a pre-heated oven at 180 degrees C (gas mark 4) for 35–40 minutes. Remove the fillets with a perforated spoon and allow to cool, then chop into large cubes.

Heat the olive oil in a large frying pan and sauté the onion and garlic for 1–2 minutes. Add the tomatoes, tomato purée, red wine, stock and mushrooms, then simmer for 6–8 minutes. Stir in the chopped basil and chicken, season to taste and simmer for a further 15 minutes.

Lightly steam the broccoli and carrots. Garnish the chicken with fresh basil leaves and serve.

Carbohydrate content per serve: **17 grams**

Chicken burritos

If time is short, you can omit the guacamole from this recipe. Remember, if you are in the active weight-loss phase of the diet, you must have no more than one slice of bread or one tortilla per day.

For 2

200 grams skinless chicken breast

25 grams butter, cubed

2 medium flour tortillas

2 tbsp tomato salsa (see page 232)

100 ml shredded sweet romaine lettuce

100 grams guacamole (see page 222)

50 grams freshly grated Emmental (or mild cheddar, such as Orkney or Bute)

freshly ground black pepper

Place the skinless chicken breasts in a shallow, oven-safe dish, top with butter cubes, cover with pierced aluminium foil and cook in the centre of a pre-heated oven at 180 degrees C (gas mark 4) for 35–40 minutes. Remove with a perforated spoon and set aside to cool, then slice thinly. If preferred, the chicken breasts can be grilled or fried, according to taste, without affecting the diet in any way.

Allow the chicken slices to cool and then mix them with the salsa.

Wrap the tortillas in aluminium foil and place in a hot oven for 1 minute. Remove from the oven, spoon the chicken salsa mixture into the centre of each tortilla, top with shredded lettuce, guacamole and freshly grated cheese of your choice (but Emmental is ideal for this recipe). Season with freshly ground black pepper, and fold the tortilla over to close.

Carbohydrate content per serve: 33–38 grams (only 8–13 grams without the tortilla)

Tarragon chicken with tomato and avocado

For 2

250–300 grams skinless chicken breast
75 ml mayonnaise (to make your own see page 135, or a
    ready-made brand)
1 tbsp chopped fresh tarragon
pinch of rock salt
freshly ground black pepper
sprigs of fresh tarragon, to garnish
tomato and avocado salad (see pages 222–23)

Bake the chicken as described on page 202, allow to cool, then slice thinly.

Stir the chopped tarragon into the mayonnaise and season to taste. Arrange the chicken slices on the plate and top with the tarragon mayonnaise. Serve with the tomato and avocado salad, garnished with sprigs of fresh tarragon.

Carbohydrate content per serve: 8 grams (including salad)

Roast duck with juniper berries and orange liqueur sauce

For 4

2 tbsp fresh juniper berries, crushed

pinch of rock salt

freshly ground black pepper

50 grams butter

1 oven-ready duck (2.5–3 kg)

150 grams carrots, julienne

150 grams yellow squash

150 grams mangetout

Sauce

50 grams unsalted butter

2 tsp cornflour

200 ml chicken stock

1 tbsp freshly squeezed lemon juice

3 tbsp freshly squeezed orange juice

1 tbsp sweet sherry

50 ml Cointreau

Mix the crushed juniper berries, salt and freshly ground black pepper in a bowl, and transfer to a plate. Rub the butter over the duck, then roll the duck in the juniper berry mixture. Prick the duck skin liberally with a skewer. Place the duck on a rack in a roasting tin to allow the excess fat to drain as the duck is cooking, and cook at 220 degrees C (gas mark 7) for 20 minutes, then reduce the heat to 180 degrees C (gas mark 4) and cook for 2½–3 hours (depending on the size of the duck), basting once. Remove from the oven and allow to cool.

Lightly steam the carrots, squash and mangetout until tender but still firm.

While the duck is cooking, prepare the sauce. Melt the butter in a small saucepan, remove from the heat and gradually stir in the cornflour to form a smooth paste. Stir in the stock to an even consistency, then return to the heat and simmer gently. Stir in the lemon juice, orange juice and sherry over a low simmer. Add the Cointreau when the sauce thickens. Remove from the heat, continuing to stir.

Carve the duck and serve with the carrots, yellow squash and mangetout, and – of course – the orange liqueur sauce.

*Carbohydrate content per serve: **21 grams***

Chapter 14

Eggs

As I have already mentioned, eggs provide many of the proteins, vitamins and minerals essential for good health. They are also an excellent source of cysteine, the amino acid essential for the production of a major antioxidant enzyme, glutathione.

Eggs can form the basis of a meal at any time of day; the following recipes can be eaten for breakfast, brunch, lunch or supper, the only difference being that some take a little longer than others, or may be more savoury. Eggs certainly don't have to be included in your diet every day – and don't have to included at all if you don't like eggs. They should only be used in one meal per day at the most – so if you've had eggs for breakfast, don't have eggs for supper.

Egg mayonnaise sandwiches

Probably the easiest way to prepare eggs for sandwiches is by hard-boiling them at breakfast, then cooling them and chopping them finely. They can be used in an almost unlimited range of combinations. A brief selection of possibilities follows.

For 2

3 large free-range eggs, hard-boiled and chopped
1 tbsp mayonnaise (home-made or commercial)
freshly ground black pepper
2 slices buttered wholemeal bread

Mix the eggs with mayonnaise, season with freshly ground black pepper and serve on buttered wholemeal bread.

Carbohydrate content per serve: 17 grams (ie the carbohydrate content of the bread; eggs and mayonnaise are virtually carbohydrate-free)

> *This basic recipe can be enhanced by the following additions:*

- diced avocado
- finely chopped vine-ripened tomato
- sliced smoked salmon
- chopped fresh basil
- sliced Lebanese cucumber and chopped fresh chives
- curly endive lettuce and chopped fresh coriander
- red and yellow peppers, deseeded and finely diced
- diced vine-ripened tomatoes with chopped fresh chives and basil
- diced green chilli and avocado

Carbohydrate content per serve: 2–3 grams

Piperade

For 2

50 grams butter
1 small red pepper, deseeded and diced
1 small yellow pepper, deseeded and diced
1 small onion, peeled and finely chopped
1 garlic clove, peeled and finely chopped
2 large fresh plum tomatoes, skinned, seeded and diced

pinch of rock salt

freshly ground black pepper

4 large free-range eggs

2 tbsp full-cream milk

1 tsp fresh coriander, finely chopped

black olives chopped, to garnish (optional)

Melt the butter and sauté the peppers, onion and garlic for about 3–4 minutes. Add the tomatoes, season to taste and cook for another 2 minutes.

Whisk the eggs with the milk and pour over the vegetables. Add the chopped coriander, stirring gently until the mixture just sets but is still creamy, and serve immediately, garnished with chopped black olives.

Carbohydrate content per serve: 7 grams

Smoked salmon with creamy eggs

This is a very rich dish. Three large eggs therefore provide a satisfying meal for two.

For 2

3 large free-range eggs

2 tbsp single cream

freshly ground black pepper

25 grams unsalted butter

50 grams smoked salmon, finely sliced

2 tsp chopped fresh dill

pinch of paprika

Beat together the eggs and 1 tablespoon of the cream, and season with freshly ground black pepper (salt is not really

necessary for this dish as smoked salmon is naturally salty).
Melt the butter in a small saucepan and scramble the eggs
lightly. When the eggs have almost set but are still creamy,
mix in the smoked salmon and the remaining cream,
gently heat through and serve on warm plates, garnished
with chopped fresh dill and a pinch of paprika.

Carbohydrate content per serve: **negligible**

Prosciutto and courgette frittata

For 2

50 grams butter

1 small onion, peeled and diced

1 garlic clove, peeled and finely chopped

1 small red pepper, deseeded and thinly sliced

1 medium courgette, thinly sliced

4 large free-range eggs

50 ml full-cream milk

pinch of rock salt

freshly ground black pepper

2 tsp Worcestershire sauce

100 grams freshly grated cheese. Italian cheeses such as
Parmesan or Fontina are ideal, but this dish can
readily adapt to individual taste. Gruyere, Emmental,
Edam or even stronger cheeses such as Wensleydale
are equally effective

pinch of rock salt

freshly ground black pepper

2 thin slices of prosciutto, finely shredded

Melt the butter in a medium frying pan and sauté the onion,

garlic and red pepper for about 2 minutes. Add the courgette, and sauté for a further 2–3 minutes, until soft but firm. Beat the eggs and milk together with the salt, freshly ground pepper and Worcestershire sauce in a bowl, then mix in 75 grams of grated cheese. Pour the mixture over the vegetables, stirring gently to cover the base of the pan with the egg mixture. Cook over a very low heat until the mixture just sets, which usually takes about 10 minutes. Sprinkle the shredded ham over the frittata, then top with grated cheese to ensure that all of the ham is covered. Place under a hot grill for about 30–40 seconds, or until the cheese has just melted. Remove from the heat, allow the frittata to cool, then remove from the pan with a palette knife and halve. Serve with crispy green salad (see pages 229–30) or rocket and avocado salad (see page 233).

Carbohydrate content per serve: 13 grams with green salad, 8 grams with rocket salad

Baked eggs with lemon cream sauce and chives

For 2

2 large free-range eggs
75 ml single cream
1 tbsp freshly squeezed lemon juice
freshly ground black pepper
1 tbsp chopped fresh chives and ground paprika, to
    garnish

Butter 2 ramekins, gently break an egg into each one and bake in a pre-heated oven at 180 degrees C (gas mark 4) for

7–8 minutes (depending on the size of the eggs).

While the eggs are baking, gently heat the cream in a small saucepan and gradually stir in the lemon juice. Season with freshly ground black pepper.

Remove the eggs from the oven, pour the lemon sauce over the eggs, and garnish with chopped chives and ground paprika. Serve with tomato and avocado salad (see pages 222–23).

Carbohydrate content per serve: **9 grams**

Chicken and pepper frittata

Frittata is so delicious cold the next day that I always make extra for additional snacks or meals.

For 4

2 chicken breasts, about 150 grams each

25 grams butter, cubed

2 tbsp extra-virgin olive oil

1 red onion, peeled and diced

1 garlic clove, peeled and finely chopped

1 small green pepper, deseeded and finely sliced

1 small yellow pepper, deseeded and finely sliced

6 large free-range eggs, beaten

pinch of rock salt

freshly ground black pepper

50 grams freshly grated Gruyere

Place the chicken breast fillets in a shallow oven-safe dish, top with cubes of butter, cover with pierced aluminium foil and cook in the centre of a pre-heated oven at 180 degrees C (gas mark 4) for 35–40 minutes. Remove the chicken with a perforated spoon, allow to cool, then slice into thin strips.

Heat the olive oil in a medium frying pan and sauté the onion and garlic for about 1 minute. Add the peppers and sauté for a further 3–4 minutes, then return the chicken to the pan, add the eggs and season to taste. Stir in the Gruyere cheese and cook over a low heat until just set. Place under the grill for 30–40 seconds to lightly brown, and serve.

Carbohydrate content per serve: **6 grams**

Scrambled eggs and asparagus

For 2

3 large free-range eggs
2 tbsp full-cream milk
25 grams butter
pinch of rock salt
freshly ground black pepper
50 grams freshly grated Jarlsberg
100 grams fresh asparagus
1 tbsp chopped fresh chives, to garnish

Scramble the eggs (see pages 82–83) until they are just beginning to set but still creamy. Season to taste, transfer to a small shallow grill-safe dish and top with freshly grated Jarlsberg cheese. Place under a hot grill until the cheese has just melted.

In the meantime, lightly steam the asparagus until just tender.

Arrange the asparagus on warm plates, top with cheesy scrambled eggs, and garnish with chopped fresh chives.

Carbohydrate content per serve: **2 grams**

Poached egg with Swiss cheese

You can vary the cheese used in this recipe according to individual taste. I prefer continental cheeses for their more delicate flavour. The protein content is the same for all.

For 2

2 large free-range eggs
50 grams of freshly grated Emmental
freshly ground black pepper
2 slices buttered wholemeal toast

Poach the eggs, then remove from the boiling water with a perforated spoon and place on a slice of hot, buttered wholemeal toast. Sprinkle with the Emmental and place under a hot grill until the cheese melts. Add freshly ground black pepper to taste.

Carbohydrate content per serve: **17 grams (or 'nil', without the toast)**

Cheesy egg tomatoes

*This dish provides a magnificently nutritious
breakfast, with calcium and protein from the
cheese; antioxidants (lycopene) and vitamins
A and C from the tomatoes; and protein,
vitamins, minerals and antioxidants from the
eggs. It can be equally successful as a light
lunch or supper dish.*

For 2

2 large beefsteak tomatoes
pinch of rock salt
1 shallot, peeled and finely diced
$1/2$ clove of garlic, peeled and finely chopped
2 large free-range eggs
50 grams grated Gouda or Edam
1 tbsp sour cream
freshly ground black pepper
1 tbsp fresh basil, finely chopped

Cut the tomatoes in half, scoop out the contents with a
teaspoon and discard. Lay the tomatoes upside down to
drain for about 10 minutes, then place them in individual
oven-safe dishes with the open end uppermost. Add a small
pinch of salt to each tomato. Mix together the shallot and
garlic, and add half to each tomato. Gently break an egg
into each tomato. Mix the sour cream with the basil, spoon
a dessert-spoonful over each egg and season with freshly
grated black pepper. Top with grated cheese and bake in
the centre of a pre-heated oven at 190 degrees C (gas mark
4) for about 15 minutes.

Carbohydrate content per serve: 6 grams

Chapter 15

Vegetable Dishes

Leeks and lemon hollandaise sauce

For 2

8 baby leeks

pinch of rock salt

freshly ground black pepper

4 tbsp lemon hollandaise sauce (see page 00)

Season the leeks and lightly steam until tender but still firm. Remove with a perforated spoon, place on warm plates and pour the sauce over.

*Carbohydrate content per serve: **6 grams***

Char-grilled vegetables with oregano

For 2

1 medium red pepper, deseeded and chopped into large
   pieces

1 medium yellow pepper, deseeded and chopped into
   large pieces

6 baby onions, peeled and halved

1 courgette, sliced lengthways

6 cherry tomatoes

2 tbsp extra-virgin olive oil

pinch of rock salt

freshly ground black pepper

fresh oregano leaves to garnish

Dressing

4 tbsp extra-virgin olive oil

1 tbsp balsamic vinegar

1 tsp freshly squeezed lemon juice

2 tsp chopped fresh oregano

freshly ground black pepper

Place the dressing ingredients in a screw-top jar and shake until thoroughly mixed.

Arrange the vegetables in a single layer, skin uppermost, on a shallow grill-safe buttered baking tray, brush with extra-virgin olive oil and grill under medium heat for 5–6 minutes, turning frequently. Remove from the grill, peel the skin from the peppers and onion, and transfer to warm plates. Drizzle the dressing over the vegetables, season to taste and serve garnished with fresh oregano leaves.

Carbohydrate content per serve: 8 grams

Ratatouille

For 2

1 medium aubergine, cubed

pinch of rock salt

3 tbsp extra-virgin olive oil

2 courgettes, chopped

1 medium red pepper, deseeded and chopped

1 medium yellow pepper, deseeded and chopped

1 large onion, peeled and sliced

1 garlic clove, peeled and finely chopped

3 large plum tomatoes, peeled and chopped

75 ml tomato juice

1 tbsp tomato purée

pinch of granulated sugar

1 bay leaf

1 tbsp chopped fresh basil

1 tsp chopped fresh oregano

freshly ground black pepper

fresh basil leaves, to garnish

Place the chopped aubergine into a colander, sprinkle with salt, allow to stand for 20–30 minutes, then rinse with cold water and pat dry.

Heat 2 tablespoons of the extra-virgin olive oil in a large frying pan (or preferably a wok) until hot, add the aubergine, courgettes and peppers, and sauté for 2 minutes. Remove with a perforated spoon and cover.

Heat the remaining tablespoon of olive oil in the pan and sauté the onion and garlic. Add the tomatoes, tomato juice, tomato purée, sugar and bay leaf; return the aubergine, courgettes and peppers to the pan, and stir in the basil and oregano. Season to taste and gently simmer for about 6–7 minutes. Remove the bay leaf and serve, garnished with fresh basil leaves.

*Carbohydrate content per serve: **16 grams***

Spinach and cheese 'sausages' with lemon butter

For 2

300 grams fresh spinach

200 grams ricotta

75 grams freshly grated Gruyere

1 large free-range egg, beaten

pinch of freshly grated nutmeg

2 tbsp plain flour

pinch of rock salt

freshly ground black pepper

60 grams butter

2 tsp freshly squeezed lemon juice

lime zest, to garnish

Lightly steam the spinach until softened. Allow to cool. Remove and discard the stalks, then chop the leaves finely in a blender.

Mix the spinach, the ricotta, 50 grams of the Gruyere, the egg and a pinch of nutmeg in a large bowl, and season to taste. Form a malleable dough, then mould the mixture into 6–7-cm 'sausages' and roll them in the flour. Add the sausages to a large pan of boiling, salted water, cook for approximately 2 minutes and remove with a perforated spoon.

Whilst the sausages are cooking, melt the butter in a saucepan, stir in the lemon juice and season to taste. Serve the sauce over the sausages and sprinkle over the remaining grated Gruyere. Place under a medium grill until the cheese just melts, and serve, garnished with lime zest.

*Carbohydrate content per serve: **16 grams***

Asparagus with mustard hollandaise sauce

For 2

100 grams fresh asparagus, trimmed
freshly ground black pepper
1 tbsp chopped fresh chives

Sauce

Prepare the hollandaise sauce according to the recipe on
page 131, reducing the lemon juice to 1 tsp. When
prepared, stir in 2 tsp Dijon mustard.

Lightly steam the asparagus until tender but still firm.
Arrange on warm plates. Add the mustard to the
hollandaise and pour over the asparagus. Season with
freshly ground black pepper and garnish with chopped
fresh chives.

Carbohydrate content per serve: 3 grams

Baked fennel with basil and Gruyere

For 2

3 fennel bulbs, peeled
25 grams butter, cubed
1 tbsp chopped fresh basil
pinch of rock salt
freshly ground black pepper
50 grams freshly grated Gruyere
fresh basil leaves, to garnish

Place the fennel (in a single layer) in the base of a large saucepan. Add only sufficient water to almost cover, then bring to the boil and simmer until the fennel just softens. Remove with a perforated spoon and halve the fennel bulbs lengthways. Place in the base of a shallow oven-safe dish in a single layer, and sprinkle with chopped basil and cubes of butter. Season to taste, and top with a layer of Gruyere. Bake in the centre of a pre-heated oven at 180 degrees C (gas mark 4) for 10 minutes and serve, garnished with fresh basil leaves.

*Carbohydrate content per serve: **4 grams***

Stir-fried vegetables

For 2

3 tbsp extra-virgin olive oil
1 garlic clove, peeled and finely chopped
2 slices of fresh ginger root, peeled and finely chopped
75 grams broccoli florets
3 spring onions, chopped into 4–5-cm lengths
1 medium red pepper, deseeded and finely sliced
1 medium yellow pepper, deseeded and finely sliced
100 grams mangetout
50 grams button mushrooms, wiped and halved
2 tbsp light soy sauce
2 tbsp sweet sherry
pinch of rock salt
freshly ground black pepper

Heat the olive oil in a wok, sauté the garlic and ginger for about 30 seconds, then add the broccoli, spring onions,

peppers, mangetout, mushrooms, soy sauce and sherry.
Season to taste and stir-fry over medium heat for 3–4
minutes, then serve immediately.

*Carbohydrate content per serve: **12 grams***

Chapter 16

Salads

Guacamole

For 2

1 large ripe Hass avocado, halved, stoned, peeled and
  finely diced

$^1/_2$ garlic clove, peeled and finely grated

$^1/_2$ a small onion, peeled and finely chopped

$^1/_2$ ripe plum tomato, peeled, seeded and finely chopped

$^1/_2$ a fresh green chilli, deseeded and finely chopped

2 tsp freshly squeezed lime juice

1 tbsp crème fraîche

freshly ground black pepper

Blend together the avocado, garlic, onion, tomato, chilli,
lime juice and crème fraîche. Season to taste and chill
before serving.

Carbohydrate content per serve: **5 grams**

Tomato and avocado salad

For 2

1 medium, ripe Hass avocado, halved, stoned, peeled
  and diced

2 tsp freshly squeezed lemon juice

4 large vine-ripened tomatoes, chopped

1 small yellow pepper, deseeded and sliced

1 medium red onion, peeled and sliced into thin rings
freshly ground black pepper

Vinaigrette
4 tbsp extra-virgin olive oil
1 tbsp balsamic vinegar
pinch of rock salt
freshly ground black pepper

Add the virgin olive oil, balsamic vinegar, salt and freshly ground black pepper to a screw-top jar and mix thoroughly.

Mix the avocado with the lemon juice, then add the tomatoes and onion. Season to taste and drizzle the balsamic vinaigrette over the salad.

Carbohydrate content per serve: **8 grams**

Feta salad

For 2
$1/2$ a cos lettuce, washed and leaves separated
3 plum tomatoes, chopped
3 spring onions, chopped into 4–5-cm lengths
1 small Lebanese cucumber, sliced lengthways
1 small yellow pepper, deseeded and sliced
50 grams feta cheese, cubed
25 grams black olives

Vinaigrette
4 tbsp extra-virgin olive oil
1 tbsp white wine vinegar

pinch of rock salt

freshly ground black pepper

Mix the salad ingredients in a large bowl.

Place the olive oil, white wine vinegar, salt and freshly ground black pepper in a screw-top jar and mix thoroughly. Toss the salad and drizzle the dressing over.

Carbohydrate content per serve: **16 grams**

Avocado and mint sauce

A warning! For this recipe do not prepare the avocado before you make the sauce, or it will discolour. Freshly prepared with lime juice it will remain an attractive green.

For 2

1 medium, ripe Hass avocado, halved, stoned, peeled and diced

2 tsp freshly squeezed lime juice

100 ml sour cream

1 tbsp chopped fresh mint

pinch of rock salt

freshly ground black pepper

sprigs of fresh mint and lime wedges to garnish

Purée the avocado with the lime juice. Mix in the sour cream and chopped fresh mint, and season to taste. Cover and chill for at least 2 hours before serving, garnished with sprigs of fresh mint and lime wedges.

Carbohydrate content per serve: **4 grams**

Tomato and coriander salsa

For 2

4 large plum tomatoes, chopped

3 spring onions, finely chopped

$1/2$ a small green chilli, deseeded and finely chopped

1 tbsp chopped fresh coriander

pinch of rock salt

freshly ground black pepper

vinaigrette (see page 223)

sprigs of fresh coriander, to garnish

Mix together the tomatoes, onion, chilli and chopped coriander, and season to taste. Drizzle the vinaigrette over the salsa and garnish with fresh coriander.

Carbohydrate content per serve: **7 grams**

Rocket and olive salad

For 2

Handful of rocket leaves

8–10 green olives

1 tbsp freshly squeezed lemon juice

1 tbsp macadamia nut oil

25 grams freshly shaved Parmesan

freshly ground black pepper

Mix the rocket leaves and green olives. Drizzle the lemon juice and nut oil over the salad, garnish with freshly shaved Parmesan and season with freshly ground black pepper.

Carbohydrate content per serve: **1 gram**

Courgette and sour cream with basil

For 2

2 courgettes, halved, then sliced lengthways into
   matchsticks

12 mangetout, halved on the diagonal

1 green pepper, deseeded and thinly sliced

pinch of rock salt

lime zest and fresh basil leaves, to garnish

Dressing

100 ml sour cream

I garlic clove, peeled and grated

1 tbsp chopped fresh basil leaves

1 tsp freshly squeezed lime juice

Mix together the sour cream, garlic, chopped fresh basil
and lime juice, cover and chill in the fridge for 2–3 hours.

Lightly steam the courgettes, mangetout and green
pepper, allow to cool, then top with the basil and sour
cream dressing, and garnish with the lime zest and fresh
basil leaves.

*Carbohydrate content per serve: **8 grams***

Bocconcini and avocado salad

For 2

2 cherry tomatoes

1 small ripe Hass avocado, halved, stoned, peeled and
   finely sliced

100 grams Bocconcini cheese, finely sliced

freshly ground black pepper

1 tbsp chopped fresh basil leaves
balsamic vinaigrette (see page 223)

Place a cherry tomato in the centre of each plate and arrange the slices of avocado around the tomato like the spokes of a wheel. Arrange the Bocconcini slices on the avocado, season with freshly ground black pepper, garnish with chopped basil leaves and drizzle the balsamic vinaigrette over the salad.

*Carbohydrate content per serve: **2 grams***

Tomato and Parmesan salad

For 2
6 large plum tomatoes, chopped into big chunks
8 black olives
freshly ground black pepper
1 tbsp chopped fresh chives
balsamic vinaigrette (see page 223)
75 grams freshly grated Parmesan
sprigs of fresh basil, to garnish

Mix together the chopped tomatoes and olives, and place on a shallow dish. Season with freshly ground black pepper and sprinkle the chopped fresh chives over. Drizzle over the dressing, sprinkle with freshly grated Parmesan, and garnish with sprigs of fresh basil.

*Carbohydrate content per serve: **9 grams***

Radish and basil salad

For 2

4 radishes, thinly sliced

1 Lebanese cucumber, diced

1 tbsp chopped fresh chives

1 tbsp chopped fresh basil

2 tsp freshly squeezed lime juice

150 ml sour cream

pinch of rock salt

freshly ground black pepper

lime wedges

lime zest, to garnish

Mix together the radishes, cucumber, chives, basil, lime juice and sour cream in a medium bowl, season to taste and chill for at least 2 hours. Serve chilled, with lime wedges and garnished with lime zest.

Carbohydrate content per serve: 5 grams

Char-grilled pepper salad with herb mayonnaise

For 2

1 medium red pepper, deseeded and quartered

1 medium green pepper, deseeded and quartered

1 medium yellow pepper, deseeded and
   quartered

1 red onion, peeled and quartered

1 fennel bulb, peeled and quartered

2 tbsp extra-virgin olive oil

handful of red oak leaf lettuce leaves

fresh coriander leaves, to garnish

Herb mayonnaise
1 tbsp chopped fresh thyme
1 tbsp chopped fresh parsley
1 tsp chopped fresh coriander
100 ml mayonnaise (see page 135)

Mix the chopped fresh parsley and thyme into the mayonnaise.

Place the peppers (skin uppermost), onion and fennel bulb in a single layer on a grill tray. Brush with olive oil and cook under a pre-heated grill for about 5 minutes, or until the skin of the peppers blisters. Peel the peppers and remove the outer skin of the onion and fennel, then slice them into thin strips and allow to cool. Arrange the vegetables on a bed of red oak leaf lettuce leaves in a shallow dish, top with the herb mayonnaise and garnish with fresh coriander leaves.

Carbohydrate content per serve: 11 grams

Crispy green salad
For 2
100 grams mixed crispy lettuce leaves (cos, curly
   endive, coral, green oak leaf, and mizuna)
1 medium Lebanese cucumber, sliced lengthways
1 celery stick, chopped on the diagonal
1 small green pepper, deseeded and thinly sliced
1 small ripe Hass avocado, halved, stoned and diced
fresh basil leaves, to garnish

Dressing

4 tbsp extra-virgin olive oil

1 tbsp white wine vinegar

freshly ground black pepper

pinch of sugar

1 tsp Dijon mustard

Place the dressing ingredients in a screw-top jar and mix well.

Toss the green salad in a large salad bowl and pour the dressing over. Garnish with fresh basil.

Carbohydrate content per serve: 6 grams

Tomatoes and Mozzarella with mango dressing

For 2

2 large vine-ripened tomatoes, thickly sliced

100 grams of Mozzarella, sliced

slices of mango and lime zest, to garnish

Dressing

4 tbsp extra-virgin olive oil

1 tbsp white wine vinegar

2 slices fresh mango, puréed

$1/2$ tsp sesame seeds

pinch of rock salt

freshly ground black pepper

Place the dressing ingredients in a screw-top jar and shake well.

Place slices of tomato and Mozarella alternately around the circumference of a plate, and drizzle over the dressing. Garnish with slices of mango and lime zest.

Carbohydrate content per serve: **5 grams**

Cucumber and bean sprout salad

For 2

50 grams bean sprouts
1 Lebanese cucumber, sliced lengthways julienne-style
1 yellow pepper, deseeded and very thinly sliced
handful of rocket leaves
2 tbsp chopped fresh chives

Dressing

4 tbsp extra-virgin olive oil
1 tbsp balsamic vinegar
1 tsp Dijon mustard
pinch of granulated sugar
freshly ground black pepper

Place the ingredients of the dressing in a screw-top jar and shake well. Toss the salad and drizzle the dressing over. Garnish with chopped chives.

Carbohydrate content per serve: **4 grams**

Tomato salsa

For 2

4 large vine-ripened tomatoes, seeded and finely
   chopped

1 medium red onion, peeled and diced

1 garlic clove, peeled and grated

1 green chilli, deseeded, and finely chopped

1 tbsp chopped fresh basil

1 tbsp chopped fresh coriander

1 tbsp extra-virgin olive oil

Mix together the ingredients in a medium bowl, cover and
chill.

*Carbohydrate content per serve: **8 grams***

Cucumber and mint sour-cream salad

For 2

1 Lebanese cucumber, diced

3 spring onions, finely chopped

1 garlic clove, peeled and finely chopped

150 ml sour cream

1 tsp freshly squeezed lemon juice

1 tbsp chopped fresh chives

1 tbsp chopped fresh mint

pinch of rock salt

freshly ground black pepper

sprigs of fresh mint and lime zest, to garnish

Mix together the ingredients of the salad in a medium bowl, season to taste and chill in the fridge for 1–2 hours. Serve chilled, garnished with sprigs of fresh mint and lime zest.

Carbohydrate content per serve: 6 grams

Rocket and avocado salad

For 2

1 large handful of rocket leaves
1 tbsp chopped fresh basil
1 tbsp chopped fresh coriander
1 ripe Hass avocado, halved, stoned, peeled and cubed

Dressing

4 tbsp extra-virgin olive oil
1 tbsp white wine vinegar
$^1/_2$ tsp Dijon mustard
pinch of rock salt
freshly ground black pepper

Place the olive oil, white wine vinegar, mustard and seasoning in a screw-top jar and mix thoroughly. Toss the salad, and drizzle the dressing over.

Carbohydrate content per serve: 2 grams

Cucumber and chive salad

For 2

2 Lebanese cucumbers, peeled and chopped into cubes

1 tbsp chopped fresh flat leaf parsley

1 tbsp chopped fresh chives

balsamic vinaigrette (see page 223)

pinch of rock salt

freshly ground black pepper

Mix together the cucumber, parsley and chives. Drizzle the dressing over the salad and season to taste.

Carbohydrate content per serve: 1 gram

Tomato, ginger and orange salad

For 2

4 large vine-ripened tomatoes, cubed

1 large sweet orange, peeled

1 tbsp extra-virgin olive oil

2 tsp ginger wine

freshly ground black pepper

fresh basil leaves, to garnish

Divide the orange into segments, remove all the centre pith and pips, and chop into small 2–3-cm segments. Add the tomato segments, drizzle over 1 tbsp of virgin olive oil and 2 tsp of ginger wine, and mix thoroughly. Chill for at least 30 minutes, season with freshly ground black pepper and garnish with fresh basil leaves.

Carbohydrate content per serve: 11 grams

PART III

How to Exercise – Without Really Trying

Every diet book should have a chapter devoted to exercise – because even a moderate amount of regular exercise produces immense benefits for our general health – but this programme is probably going to be very different from any other you have encountered. It's not going to involve weights, complicated aerobic exercises, any special equipment, or even require much time in your busy schedule.

Chapter 17

Why Exercise

Do you *have* to exercise when you are on this diet? The answer is no, you don't *have* to exercise, because you *will* lose body fat on this diet without exercise, and you won't lose much fat from exercise alone unless you exercise for long periods every day – which has the double disadvantage of stimulating hunger (so you need to eat more food) and also stimulating the production of more insulin, which then converts the extra food into fat! Now you begin to understand why it is very difficult to lose weight by exercise alone and how it is virtually impossible to exercise on a low-calorie diet. However, you don't need to do much exercise to achieve *dramatic* changes in your physical appearance when exercise is taken in association with a diet that specifically removes body fat and leaves body musculature intact.

If you really don't want to do any exercise, I have to be honest and say that you don't have to exercise if you only want to lose fat. In other words, you will lose fat and be much slimmer on this diet without specific exercise routines. So if you really are opposed to exercise, read no further.

But with just a little time (less than 15 minutes per day) devoted to easy exercises – which almost *anyone* can do, no matter how out of condition or overweight – you can improve the *shape* of your body and look much more attractive. To understand how you can change the shape of your body in this way, I have to explain a little about anatomy – or the structural make-up of the body – in simple terms. I keep repeating that most of medicine is essentially applied common sense, and you will soon realise how true this is.

The body has an underlying framework made up of bone, – the skeleton. This is the scaffolding that supports us. Over the skeleton is a layer of muscle, then a layer of fat and finally the outer covering of skin. So you can easily appreciate that if you reduce the fat layer, you will become slimmer, but if you also – even slightly – tighten or tone-up the muscle layer, you will *suddenly assume a smooth, toned body shape*.

Rather than just being thinner, you will be slimmer *with shape* as a result of the increased muscle tone.

Achieving this attractive body shape does not need to involve complex weight training or exhausting, prolonged aerobic exercises, but rather *a simple series of specially designed exercises which you can perform in the privacy of your own home without expensive equipment*.

Let us return to the primary reason for being on a diet – simply because, like most people, you want to look better, slimmer and more attractive. And if you succeed, you assume – probably correctly – that you will have more self-confidence. So, surely, if you lose fat you'll look better, feel better and probably have elevated self-esteem and therefore self-confidence. You might think, why bother exercising? It all comes back to the body shape to which you aspire. By that I don't want to give any false impression that I can transform you into a supermodel, but with just a *little* exercising to improve the *tone* of your body, you will reveal the contoured shape of the real you. And it is much better than you think! We can't change our inherent genetic characteristics, but we can definitely change the amount of fat we are carrying around with us. If your muscles are flabby (and they probably are), without exercise you will be slimmer but still a little shapeless.

If, however, you perform 10–15 minutes per day of *very* light exercise – and I mean *very* light – which can be done in your own home at any time of day (without embarrassment) – you will quickly tone up your muscles, and as the fat drops away, you will be left with a much more attractive body shape – with very little effort!

The ultimate underlying purpose of this book is really to demonstrate that you *can* lose your excess fat, tone up your muscles, look great and feel great with *no pain and very little effort*. You will look and feel much better on this integrated programme *within 2 weeks,* although obviously it will take some time to lose all the excess fat at 1–1¹/₂ kilos per week, depending on how much there is to lose. All those years of struggling to lose weight are over!

The other major importance of exercise is that it improves circulation. Even a little exercise opens the tiny blood vessels, called capillaries, in all the tissues of the body, so the tissues receive more oxygen and nutrition. The better the circulation of blood around the body, the easier it is to remove the waste products of cells in the body. I don't intend to give a technical explanation of the mechanisms of blood circulation – which is of little interest to the reader who only wishes to lose weight as fat. The bottom line is that with improved circulation and the associated cleansing of cellular waste products *we feel much better*.

And at the end of the day, that's the whole purpose of this diet: to make you look better and feel better.

Now to the exercise 'regime'. There's really no 'regime' at all, and you will be amazed at how easy it is to alter your body shape *medically*. This is really the difference between this programme of exercise and diet, and others that have been published; this is based on established medical principles, whereas some others seem to be little more than the fad of the moment.

First, we have to dispel some common myths about exercise and weight loss:

• *Exercise burns fat*

No, it doesn't! Of course, if you exercise for long periods, it is theoretically possible to burn off fat – but you have to exercise regularly for extended periods (which is virtually impossible for most people) and it also makes the ridiculous assumption that, after considerable aerobic exercise, you then have the will-power to ignore the ravenous hunger *induced by the exercise*. Perhaps some people can perform this minor miracle, but not many!

• *No pain, no gain*

Absolute rubbish! In fact, worse than rubbish, it's clinically dangerous. If you are overweight and you exercise to the point of inducing pain, the next pain you are likely to experience is that of a coronary thombosis. In people unaccustomed to regular exercise, exercise must be used only for its primary purpose of toning up the muscles and improving the circulation. This is sufficient to produce a significant improvement in body shape, and actually reduces the risk of a heart attack – with a relatively low level of exercise.

- *You have to exercise for at least an hour per day, three times per week, for it to be effective*

Not true! I will shortly be describing isometric exercises which will tone up your muscles and improve circulation in a few minutes per day. Of course, additional aerobic exercise, in particular walking, is very beneficial. I would advise walking 10–15 minutes per day (which is most easily achieved by either alighting from the bus one stop away from work or parking a little further away).

To exercise properly, you really need to understand a few technical terms. By understanding the *purpose* of what you are doing – which, once again, is very simple – you take control of your own body. Always remember, it's your body, nobody will take as much care of it as you, and armed with the requisite knowledge you can be as healthy as you want to be. The concept of effective exercise is *very* easy, and once you understand the concepts, you will never again be fooled by some of the so-called experts whose only purpose seems to be making a significant proportion of the overweight population feel guilty because they are unable to exercise like Olympic athletes!

Exercise can be **aerobic** or **anaerobic**. **Aerobic** exercise simply means that we take in sufficient oxygen to burn off energy as we exercise. **Anaerobic** exercise is the opposite: we *don't* take in enough oxygen for the exercise, as in sprinting, for example. When you exercise *anaerobically*, your body tells you to stop by giving you pain (from the build-up of a substance called 'lactic acid' in the muscles). So you can now understand why you should **never** experience pain during exercise; it means there is insufficient oxygen for the muscles to perform the exercise in progress. *This it is not necessary for effective exercise, in fact it is positively undesirable.*

All of the exercise we perform must be **aerobic**, where we can easily absorb all of the oxygen we need during the activity: in other words, *no pain*. Incidentally, this is *not* the same as *aerobics*, which is just a play on the word 'aerobic'. 'Aerobics' are simply movement exercises, which if too severe may become 'anaerobic' – in other words, they cause pain!

The only other fact you need to know about exercise is that it can be either **isotonic** or **isometric**. This sounds very technical, but it's not; once again, it's very easy to understand. **Isotonic** exercises are those which we immediately think of when the word 'exercise' is mentioned. They involve muscles actually moving: running, lifting, stepping and stretching. In other words, all of the exercises overweight people dislike because they can't do them, and it's embarrassing to try in front of others! The obvious conclusion is that these are *not* the best forms of exercise for the overweight, so isotonic exercises – apart from walking, which is the best and safest isotonic exercise by far – are not included in this programme. If you wish, you can commence isotonic exercises after your muscles have increased tone and you have lost weight, but it is not essential.

Of course, all forms of exercise – in moderation – can be beneficial, and if you are currently following a particular exercise regime, continue that programme. But you should be aware that jogging and aerobics can be detrimental to knee and hip joints in those who are significantly overweight, and may have adverse cardiac (heart) implications if you commence these strenuous exercises over-enthusiastically for the first time.

The other major category of exercise – which is appropriate because it can be easily performed by *everyone* – is **isometric** exercise. In this well-established form of exercise, **muscles do not move**. That is correct, you exercise *without actually moving*.

First of all, I tell you that your body fat will *automatically* begin reducing if you cut out refined carbohydrates from your diet – but you can eat virtually unlimited amounts of other foods – and now I am telling you that you can exercise, to become much stronger and with a significant improvement in body shape – *without moving*! No, I haven't lost my senses, and this is true. In fact, it is a technique routinely used by many athletes in their training programme.

Isometric exercise is based upon the concept that a muscle will develop its maximal power *at its resting length*, which essentially means *without moving but at maximum tension*.

What does that mean in practice? The most effective way to explain the concept is for you to perform one of these simple exercises whilst you are sitting reading this book – *but before commencing any exercise programme, you **must** consult your doctor first*. Exercising when you are overweight can be very dangerous unless performed under careful medical supervision. Isometric exercise can increase blood pressure (and all exercise will increase blood pressure to some degree); therefore **isometric exercise should not be performed by patients with high blood pressure or heart disease.** If you fall into either of these categories, the most beneficial exercise would be walking 10–15 minutes per day.

Providing you have no pre-existing medical condition

which is likely to be made worse by unaccustomed exercise, and you have been given the all clear by your doctor, you can proceed with the exercise programme. Remember, you will become slimmer on the diet alone. The exercise programme I am about to describe will merely improve the shape of your slimmer body; it won't actually make you slimmer in itself. So if it's not safe for you to exercise – *don't!* I am first and foremost a physician, which means that I will always advise caution: never take risks with your health!

Let us proceed with an exercise which will clearly demonstrate how easily you can alter your body shape (for the better) in a few minutes per day, and wherever you may be. Place both hands in front of you, elbows bent, palms together, about 15 cm from your chest.

Chest muscle exercise

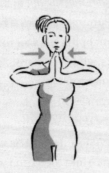

Now, take a moderate breath in and, whilst holding your breath, press both palms against one another *as hard as you can* for 8–10 seconds, then relax. You have just performed one of the major exercises for strengthening the muscles of the chest (the pectoral muscles). You can probably feel a tightening of the chest muscles already. If you perform this exercise on a daily basis – only 8–10 seconds of continuous exercise – you will strengthen these muscles, and in the process they will assume a smooth contour. As you lose the overlying layer of fat, the body shape underneath will assume a firm, attractive contour, rather than being flabby.

Women need not worry about developing a too muscular body. The beauty of this form of exercise is that it tones muscles but does not create a masculine contour. You will be even more feminine with muscular tone, particularly in 'difficult' areas such as the upper arms. In this part of the female anatomy, excess accumulation of fat cells, in association with poor muscle tone, causes the characteristic appearance of 'dimpled' skin. The diet will reduce the fat layer, and the isometric exercises will increase muscle tone, producing a smoother, firmer upper arm.

Remember, women have a thicker fat layer over their bodies than males, which gives the female form a smoother contour, without muscles 'bulging' out, as in the typical (but rarely seen!) muscular male body shape.

Although this genetically inherited fat layer may seem a disadvantage, it certainly is not; you can use it to your advantage in shaping your body contour. If you diet *properly*, you will retain the underlying muscles, whilst losing some – but not all – of the overlying fat layer. If you then increase the tone of those muscles, their even contour will smooth out the lax overlying skin, removing to a large degree the unsightly dimpling that is sometimes called cellulite.

This rationale works equally successfully for men. You simply use the genetically determined pattern for the shape of your body. What does all this mean? In simple terms, the male body is programmed by its genes to have a thinner fat layer over the muscles than the female. So if you remove the fat, by diet, and increase the tone of the muscles, by isometric exercise, you return to the natural male body shape, with the muscles obvious under a thinner fat layer.

It seems remarkably simple, because it is! The secret is to employ a proper diet and exercise programme to return the body to its natural shape.

If you use the *wrong* diet, and lose protein instead of fat, you will still be thinner, but you cannot then sculpt the body because you don't have any muscles left to sculpt! And if you use the *wrong* exercise programme, you will probably *build* excess muscle, which is often considered unattractive in a woman.

So you can clearly see that correct diet and appropriate exercise will significantly improve body shape *with very little effort or will-power*, and is equally effective in both men and women, because your body is already programmed (through your genes) to assume a particular shape. You are merely returning it to its natural shape by using the *correct* system of exercise and diet.

You can now understand the importance of *effective* dieting. In other words, you reduce *body fat* not *body bulk*: in the former, body protein is saved and body fat is selectively removed, leaving the muscle intact; in the latter, the *size* is reduced, but at the expense of muscle *(or body protein)* rather than *fat*. If planned correctly, an effective diet combined with an appropriate isometric exercise programme will reduce the outer layer of fat and accentuate the underlying muscle.

Of course, we have to exercise *all* of the different

muscle groups individually. Our bodies work by having one group of muscles perform one action (for example, moving your leg forward) and another group performing the opposite action (moving the leg backward). If you only exercise the first group, you will become unbalanced in muscular terms, so it is very important that you follow the exercise programme carefully and always exercise *two* groups of muscles on every occasion, the **agonist** and the **antagonist**. Medical terms, but very simple. An 'agonist' is a muscle that moves your body in one direction (for example, bending the arm), and an 'antagonist' is a muscle that moves it in the opposite direction (straightening the arm).

Whenever you exercise an 'agonist' in one direction, you always have to exercise the 'antagonist' muscle in the opposite direction to keep in balance, it's as simple as that. By exercising all of the muscle groups individually, you will achieve an evenly balanced, firm toning of the body, and the whole exercise programme will take no more than 10 minutes per day. These exercises can be performed in the home, at the office or even in the car, whilst waiting in traffic – without you appearing 'odd' to adjacent drivers!

This exercise programme is safer than many others *because you are exercising against yourself*. You are *not* lifting heavy weights, with all the attendant risks involved, or stretching muscles and joints that haven't experienced a wide range of movement for years. In isometric exercise, one half of the body is exercising against the other half, which keeps the body in equal balance, and as you only exert as much effort as you are able, *you* are always in total control of the level of exertion. This is very important because many accidents occur with unaccustomed exercise involving over-exertion with exercise equipment. With isometric exercise, the exercise 'equipment' is your own body!

A comprehensive series of balanced exercises follows. Please follow the recommended exercise programme without omitting any of the exercises, because deviation from the programme could result in an imbalance of muscular power. For example, if you perform the exercise for the front of the arm (to tighten the skin over dimples of cellulite) *without* exercising the rear part of the arm, you will have an imbalance between bending and straightening the arm. Providing you always remember to exercise both the *agonist* muscle and its *antagonist* muscle, which is clearly explained in the table on page 266, you will have no problems.

This daily programme will give you a balanced, toned musculature, in only a little more time than it takes to make a pot of tea!

Chapter 18

An isometric exercise programme

The easiest way of ensuring that you don't miss out any of the main muscle groups when exercising is to start from the head and work down to the toes. Because if you want to look good, your muscle tone has to be balanced from head to foot.

All isometric exercises are performed whilst holding your breath, after inhaling to about half to two-thirds lung capacity, for about 8–10 seconds (the duration of each individual exercise).

The other important point to remember – and I will deliberately repeat this on several occasions because it is very important – is to **take your time** and **rest** during unaccustomed exercise. This whole programme of exercise will take less than four minutes of actual exertion, but I want you to rest for 10–20 seconds between each movement, giving a total time of 10–12 minutes, including resting periods. If you feel uncomfortable at any time, **stop immediately!** Go at your own pace; there is no rush.

Neck Exercises

Exercising the neck is *very* important for two main reasons:

1. *To help prevent arthritis of the neck*

The neck supports the head (fairly obvious), which is mechanically a very difficult action, because the head is relatively heavy and the neck is relatively weak.

Over a period of years, the discs *between* the bones in

the neck (vertebrae), gradually wear away at the junctions where the bones rub together.

If you strengthen your neck muscles by isometric exercise you help to prevent arthritis in the neck, which can be very distressing in later life.

2. *To improve the cosmetic appearance of the neck*

For most people this is the most important reason for exercising the neck. As you know, when you are on a diet there is a tendency for large, unsightly 'craters' to appear in the neck between the muscles where the fat has gone, leaving an undesirable scrawny look. If you simply increase the bulk of the muscle, you will reduce the size of the 'craters', producing a vast improvement in cosmetic appearance.

Isometric Neck Exercises

The basis of all isometric exercise is that you press *against resistance* for a period of 8–10 seconds. The resistance is provided by other muscles in the body. Neck exercises perform two main movements: forwards/backwards and lateral (side-to-side) movements.

1. *Forward/backward isometric neck exercises*

Take a deep breath in and hold. Place both hands on the front of your forehead and press your head forwards against your hands as hard as you can.

You should simultaneously press your hands against your forehead, so that there is no movement of your head. Hold this position for 8–10 seconds, then release, breathing in as you relax.

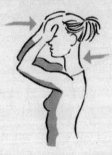

To counterbalance the effect of strengthening these muscles, you must exercise the antagonist group of muscles. Take a deep breath in, place your hands around the back of your head and press your head back against your hands, holding your head motionless by simultaneously pressing forwards with your hands. Hold for 8–10 seconds and release.

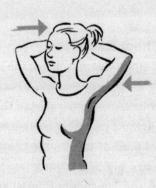

2. *Lateral isometric neck exercises*

Take a deep breath in and hold. Place the palm of your right hand on the right hand side of your head.

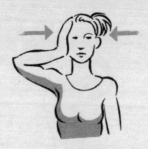

Press your head firmly against your hand, resisting the head movement by pressing your hand against your head with equal force. Hold steadily for 8–10 seconds, and release.

Repeat the exercise using the left hand against the left side of the head and hold for 8–10 seconds.

As you can see, these exercises are much harder than you would expect from a contraction of only 8–10 seconds, and you can probably feel the muscle power increasing already.

Isometric Chest Exercises

We need to exercise the muscles of the upper chest and the corresponding muscles of the upper back because this gives the rounded tone to the upper part of the body that prevents us having a pear-shaped appearance. In a woman these exercises provide tone in the chest musculature under the breasts, giving a slightly increased bust measurement, and, most importantly, an improved *shape* to the bust. However, you will not gain an overly muscular appearance (as normally associated with exercise) because of the slightly thicker overlying fat layer in women.

Place both hands, elbows bent, palms together,

approximately 15 cm in front of your chest. Breathe in to about half lung capacity, press both palms together as firmly as you can, hold the contraction for 8–10 seconds whilst holding your breath, and release.

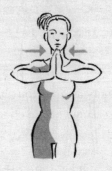

You will feel a tightening of the chest muscles and within a few weeks, these muscles will be much stronger.

As always, we have to balance one group of muscles with their antagonists. The antagonist muscles to the chest are the upper back. To exercise these muscles isometrically, stand with your back to a dining chair (or similar), place both hands behind your back and grasp the respective sides of the chair with both hands.

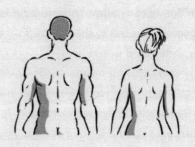

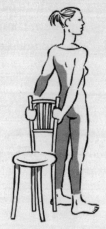

Take a deep breath in and hold. Press both hands against one another as hard as you can for 8–10 seconds and release, breathing in as you relax.

Isometric Upper Arm Exercises

Toning of the upper arm muscles is cosmetically important for both men and women, for different reasons.

When a woman increases the tone of her muscles, the thicker overlying fat layer ensures a smooth contour to the upper arm, which produces a more cosmetically attractive appearance, removing the undesirable appearance of cellulite. In a man, reduction of the naturally thinner fat layer leads to the desired muscular contour to the biceps. The net result for both sexes is a well-toned upper arm.

We begin by increasing the tone of the *flexor* muscles (biceps). Put your hands by your side. Bend your left arm up to form a right angle, keeping your elbow level with your waist. Your arm should be in a similar position to when you shake someone's hand. Place your right hand

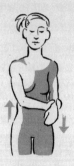

over your left wrist and grasp it. Take a deep breath in and hold. Press *up* with your left arm while resisting the movement with your right hand. The left arm should not move during the period of flexion against resistance. Hold the tension for 8–10 seconds, and relax.

Repeat the movement on the right side to exercise the right biceps, once again ensuring that your right elbow stays level with your waist. Your right arm should not move during the exercise.

Obviously, having exercised the *flexor* muscles (biceps) of the arm (which bend it), we have to exercise the *extensor* muscles (triceps) of the arm (which straighten it) to maintain a muscular balance.

Once again, bend your left arm to a right angle, but this time place your right hand *under* your left wrist, before

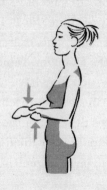

grasping it. Take a deep breath in and hold. Press *down* with your left arm whilst resisting the movement with your right arm. Hold the tension for 8–10 seconds, and relax.

Repeat the movement on the right side to exercise the right triceps. Hold the tension for 8–10 seconds, and then relax.

Isometric Shoulder Exercises

The shoulders give the upper body – both male and female – its characteristic shape. The commonest mistake in exercising is to concentrate on the chest and waist, which, although important muscle groups, do not improve the body shape unless you increase shoulder muscle tone. Think about this carefully: if you improve the tone of the shoulder muscles, your posture immediately improves, accentuating the whole body profile. Otherwise, all of your hard work to improve your appearance is undermined by droopy shoulders.

There are several groups of muscles around the shoulder joint, and we can exercise most of them in a total of less than 1 minute!

First, stand in an open doorway and place both hands, palm upwards, against the upper lintel. Take a deep breath in, hold your breath, and press upwards as hard as you can against the upper lintel for 8–10 seconds, then relax and breathe normally. This exercises the muscles on the upper part of the shoulder. Depending on the height of the doorway, you may have to stand on your toes (or possibly a small stool) to reach the lintel, but don't worry, this serves the dual purpose of exercising the muscles on the front of your thigh and the calf at the same time, as they will be in isometric tension during the exercise. You probably never realised how much exercise you could do in 10 seconds without actually moving!

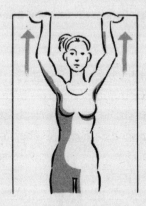

Still standing in the open doorway, make a fist with both hands and place the outer edge of each fist against the sides of the doorway. Take a deep breath in and hold your breath. Press as hard as you can against each door support for 8–10 seconds, and relax. This exercises the muscles on the outer (or lateral) part of the shoulder.

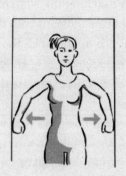

Stand facing a wall, approximately 10 cm away form it. Make a fist with both hands, place the leading edge of both fists against the wall, take a deep breath in and hold your breath. Press as hard as you can against the wall for 8–10 seconds, and relax. This exercises the muscles on the front of the shoulder.

Finally, place your back against the wall, with your

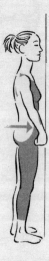

shoulders and heels touching the wall. Make a fist with both hands, place the rear edge of both fists against the wall, take a deep breath in and hold, then press back against the wall as hard as you can. Hold the tension for 8–10 seconds and relax. This exercises the muscles on the back of the shoulder.

You can now see that there are many muscle groups around the shoulder that facilitate the complex movements of the arm. We have to exercise all of these groups to maintain stability of the joint. If you exercise some and not others, you will be unbalanced. Within one week of performing these simple – but effective – shoulder muscle exercises you will feel the difference, and the best part of this form of exercising is that the more out of condition you are, the greater the improvement you feel!

One of the major advantages of *isometric* back exercises,

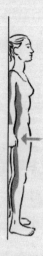

rather than the more common *isotonic* exercises, is that they allow you to strengthen your back muscles relatively safely, using only as much resistance as you consider appropriate. **However, anyone with a history of back problems must not commence an exercise programme without the approval of their family physician.**

The first exercise is very important for the latissimus dorsi, a powerful upper back muscle, which also gives a very attractive appearance to the body shape.

Sit on a chair facing a table or desk of normal height, approximately 15 cm away. Place the palms of both hands face down on the table, take a deep breath in and press down as hard as you can on the table whilst holding your breath. Hold the tension for 8–10 seconds, and relax.

The second exercise for the upper back muscles involves using a small towel, such as a tea towel. Stand upright, with feet about shoulder-width apart and your arms holding a towel about shoulder-width apart above your head.

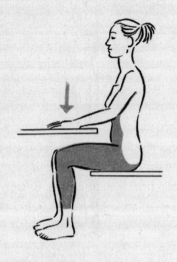

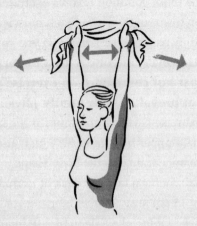

Take a deep breath in and hold. Grasp the towel tightly and try to pull both arms outwards and downwards simultaneously. Hold for 8–10 seconds, and relax.

Isometric Exercises for the Lower Back

The lower back is one of the most important parts of the body for maintaining posture, but it is also one of the main areas of weakness in many people.

Perform all back exercises with extreme caution. If you cannot sustain the contraction for 8–10 seconds, **stop immediately!** Remember, we are solving problems which have gradually developed over decades in many cases. There is *no* rush. You *will* become slimmer, stronger and fitter on the programme, but always *go at your own pace.*

Lie face down on the floor, with your arms by your sides. Take a deep breath in and hold. Raise your head and shoulders about 8–10 cm off the floor, without using your arms. Hold this position for 8–10 seconds, if possible, then relax. You will feel the tension on the lower back muscles, but if there is any discomfort, **stop immediately!**

For the second exercise, lie face down on the carpet, legs and arms extended outwards. Take a deep breath and hold. Arch your back backwards whilst trying to lift your arms and legs off the ground. Hold for 8–10 seconds, and relax.

If you cannot perform this exercise, or perhaps only for a few seconds, don't worry. It is difficult to exercise the back after years of inertia, but as your weight decreases, the exercises *will* become easier, so **do not overexert at this stage**.

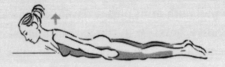

Isometric Abdominal Exercise

Like back exercises, this exercise can cause injuries, because people tend to attack it far too enthusiastically. Remember, the aim is to produce a slimmer, toned and improved body shape, not that of a professional boxer! Only perform the exercise to the level you are able, and that means if you can't do it at this stage, *don't!*

These are exercises that your are not accustomed to, and it would be *abnormal* if you *could* perform the exercises easily. You will look better with a slimmer waist from the diet, and as the fat decreases you will gradually be able to perform the abdominal exercise with ease. Do what you can, no more, and *never be afraid to stop*. No pain, no gain is for fools!

Lie flat on your back with your hands by your sides. Take a deep breath and hold, then gently lift the upper part of your body about 10 cm off the ground (using your abdominal muscles; don't push up with your hands) and hold for 8–10 seconds (or less), then relax. This is all you need to do to tighten your abdominal muscles and improve abdominal shape, *but it is a hard exercise in the beginning, so do not over-exert yourself.*

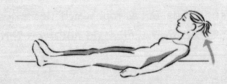

Isometric Leg Exercises

Isometric exercises for the leg muscles are relatively easy
to perform, and have the added advantage that several
groups of muscles can be exercised in the same movement.

The first exercise involves standing in an open
doorframe, with your back resting against one doorpost.
Lift one leg and place the foot against the other doorpost at
a height that is convenient to you; in other words, don't try
to lift your leg high if it is not comfortable. Take a deep
breath in and hold your breath. Brace your back against the
doorpost and press against the other doorpost as hard as
you can for 8–10 seconds, then relax. Repeat the exercise
with the other leg.

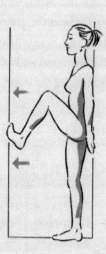

This is an excellent exercise for toning up the muscles
on the front of the thigh (quadriceps) and also the all-
important calf muscles, which give the lower leg its
contour.

Having exercised the muscles on the front of the leg, we
now have to exercise the rear of the leg (the hamstring

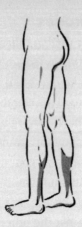

muscles) and the muscles on the bottom. Toning this area
is essential, as I am sure all will agree.

Stand with your back to a wall, both heels and shoulders
resting against the wall. Place the palms of both hands flat
against the wall for stability. Take a deep breath in and
hold, then press your right heel as hard as you can against
the wall – without propelling yourself forward – for 8–10

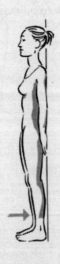

seconds, and relax. You will feel the tightening of the muscles down the back of your leg, and especially the buttock region, almost immediately.

Repeat the exercise with the left leg.

That completes the programme. Of course, I could describe isometric exercises that would improve the tone and strength of virtually every muscle group in the body, but that is not the purpose of this book. The purpose is to show you how to tone the most important muscle groups, to ensure an attractive, contoured body after removing the surface layer of fat with effective dieting. This requires only 23 exercises, each of 8–10 seconds duration, a total of 4 minutes of actual exercise. Allowing for a resting period of 20 seconds between each movement – which is double the exercise duration itself – the total time required is a maximum of 12 minutes per day. The exercises are briefly summarised in the following table.

Isometric Exercise Programme

	Agonist	Antagonist
1. **Neck**	forward movement (flexion)	backward movement (extension)
	movement to right side	movement to left side
2. **Thorax**	chest muscles	upper back muscles
3. **Shoulder**	arm movement forwards	arm movement backwards
	arm movement up	arm movement down

4. **Upper arm**	bending (flexion)	straightening (extension)
5. **Upper back**	arm movement up	arm movement down
6. **Abdomen**	abdominal muscles	lower back muscles
7. **Leg**	front leg muscles (quadriceps)	rear leg muscles (hamstrings and calf muscles)

I must emphasise that it is essential to *take it easy* when you start exercising. This programme is ideal because it is relatively easy, can be taken at your own pace, requires no special equipment and is highly effective in achieving results, but I still advise you to take your time. If you feel uncomfortable, *stop!* Remember you are still losing weight on the diet, and there is no desperate rush to increase muscle tone. Exercise must achieve its aims *gently* to be safe and effective.

At this point, it would be useful to review what this exercise programme will achieve, and also what it will not!

- If you don't diet to lose the fat, the muscles will be toned, but you won't notice them through the overlying fat layer. The exercise in itself will *not* cause significant loss of fat – but then that was never the intention.

- If you diet incorrectly, and lose protein as well as fat, you will not be able to achieve a toned body, because there is very little muscle to tone, so an appropriate *fat-losing* (not just weight-losing), *muscle-sparing* diet is essential. A high-protein, low-carbohydrate diet will achieve this desired result.

- Isometric exercise will tone and strengthen the body musculature, giving a more attractive body shape. It won't increase stamina, which can only be achieved by repetitive, time-consuming isotonic exercises (such as a treadmill), but then you don't really need this for most of normal life. If you lose fat and increase body protein, you will feel better and have more energy anyway! If you can combine these isometric exercises with a little walking (10–15 minutes per day) or swimming, you will notice a substantial improvement in your fitness level. Remember, 10–15 minutes walking is only 10 minutes to and from the bus stop or to your car, every day. It requires virtually no special arrangements or equipment to achieve. And it is medically proven to reduce risks of heart attack significantly.

Exercise of any form, especially when combined with an appropriate diet, will change your shape, but it will not attain the impossible. Be realistic and have realistic goals. Having lost all the *unnecessary* weight (as fat) and toned your muscles, you will look and feel immensely better, but it will still be you. Don't try to be someone else. The supermodels in magazines have the advantage of a photographer with an air-brush to remove any presumed cosmetic defects; it's not real life, and they don't look like that in real life!

Appendix 1:

The carbohydrate content of common snack foods

i. Foods which may be included in the diet within the 40-gram daily carbohydrate limit, with extreme caution

(Some of these items vary in size and ingredients; the carbohydrate contents are average values and can vary)

Food	Average carbohydrate content (grams of carbohydrate)
Biscuits	
(per biscuit)	
bourbon	8
chocolate coated	12
chocolate chip	7
cream	7
crunch cream	9
custard cream	8
digestive	
– plain	11
– chocolate	11
ginger nut	9
shortbread	11

Crackers and crispbreads

(per cracker/crispbread)

cream cracker	5
catcakes	6
rye crispbread	6
water biscuit	5
wholemeal cracker	5

Fruit

(per piece)

apple	13
grapefruit	10
grapes (100g)	14
kiwi fruit	10
mango (half)	12
melon (honeydew)	11
nectarine	7
orange	10
peach	9
plum	9

Nuts (per 100g)

almond	2
brazil	3
hazelnuts	6
macadamia	5
peanuts	12
pecan	6
pine	4
pistachio	8
walnut	3

Potato crisps
(per bag)

bacon and brown sauce	12
roast beef	12
roast chicken	12
tomato	12
salt	12
salt and vinegar	11
sour cream and onion	14

ii. Foods which should *not* be included in the diet
(These items vary in size and ingredients; the carbohydrate contents are average values and can vary)

Food	Average carbohydrate content (grams of carbohydrate)
Bread (each)	
bagel	30
focaccia	30
pitta	55
roll	29
sliced	15–17 (maximum of 1 slice/day)
tortilla	20–25 (maximum of 1/day)

Cake (per 100g)

apple pie	30
banana	62
cheesecake	30
chocolate	55
chocolate éclair	30
doughnut	40
Danish pastry	42
fruit	55
muffin	50
scone	46
sponge	50

Cereal (per 100g)
(examples only – *all* breakfast cereals are excluded)

muesli	72
puffed wheat	65
sultana bran	66

Fast food
(per 100 grams)
bacon and egg
  muffin

per muffin	33
cheeseburger	
per burger	35
chicken dippers	
per dipper	2
chicken nuggets	
per nugget	3
chicken, fried	
per piece (approx)	45

chips

    (oven-bake)

    per portion   72

hash brown

    per piece   15

onion bhajia

    per bhajia   4

pizza (per 100g)

    (varies)

    average pizza   33

    per slice   25

    examples:

        cheese and tomato

        (deep pan)   45

        cheese and tomato

        (thin and crispy)   28

        four cheese

        (thin and crispy)   32

        vegetable and

        Goats cheese

        (thin and crispy)   31

Quarter Pounder   20

saffron rice   24

sausage roll   25

    per roll   30

shepherd's

    pie (beef)   10

    per small pie   18

    pie (lamb)   11

    per small pie   24

potato wedges

    (oven-bake)   25

spring roll
    per roll   50
vegetable
    pakora   20
vegetable
    samosa   25

Fruit
    banana   30
    pear   19

Ice cream (100 ml)   20

Milk chocolate (per 100g)   61

Mixed nuts and raisins
    (per 100g)   32

Appendix 2:

The carbohydrate content of vegetables

i. Vegetables included without restriction in the diet

Vegetable (100g)	Average carbohydrate content (grams of carbohydrate)
Asparagus (fresh)	2
Avocado	2
Aubergine	2
Beans (French)	3
Bamboo shoots	6
Broccoli	1
Brussels sprouts	2
Cabbage	2
Carrots	7
Cauliflower	2
Celery	2
Courgettes	2
Cucumber	3
Garlic (per clove)	less than 1
Kale	5
Lettuce	2
Mushrooms (button)	2
Onions	4
Parsley	less than 1
Peas	7

Peppers:

green	2.5
red	4
yellow	4
Pumpkin	7
Radish	2
Spinach	1
Tomatoes	3
Turnips	2
Swede	2

ii. Vegetables excluded from the diet during the weight-loss phase

Vegetable (100g)	Average carbohydrate content (grams of carbohydrate)
Beetroot	14
Chickpeas	16
Corn (cob)	12
Haricot beans	18
Kidney beans	12
Lentils	17
Parsnips	13
Potatoes	
boiled	14
chipped	36
Sweet potato	21
Yam	38

Appendix 3:

The carbohydrate content of alcoholic beverages

Beverage	Average carbohydrate content (grams of carbohydrate)
Beer (1 pint)	13
Sherry (50 ml)	
dry	less than 1
sweet	4
Spirits (50 ml)	
brandy	0
gin	0
vodka	0
whisky	0
Wine (100 ml)	
white	
dry	less than 1
medium	4
sweet	6
red	less than 1

Index